ILLUSTRATED CASE HISTORIES

Cardiovascular Medicine

David H Roberts MD, MRCP

Consultant in Cardiology
Victoria Hospital
Blackpool, UK

John West MD, MRCP

Lecturer in Cardiovascular Medicine
Department of Cardiovascular Medicine
Queen Elizabeth Hospital
Birmingham, UK

William A Littler MD, FRCP

Professor of Cardiovascular Medicine
Department of Cardiovascular Medicine
Queen Elizabeth Hospital
Birmingham, UK

M Wolfe

Copyright © 1994 Mosby–Year Book Europe Limited
Published in 1994 by Wolfe Publishing, an imprint of Mosby–Year Book Europe Limited

Printed by in Spain by Grafos, S. A. Arte sobre papel

ISBN 0 7234 1935 3

For full details of all Mosby–Year Book Europe Limited titles please write to Mosby–Year Book Europe Limited, Lynton House, 7–12 Tavistock Square, London WC1H 9LB, England.

A CIP catalogue record for this book is available from the British Library.

Library of Congress Cataloging-in-Publication Data has been applied for

Contents

Preface

Cardiology is a specialty in which sophisticated technology plays an increasingly prominent role. This, of course, should not detract from the importance of basic clinical skills. We have attempted to link these two aspects into the case histories described and illustrated herewith. All the illustrations are photographs of original investigations of clinical cases. Some represent common cardiology conditions while others are rarieties. This book should therefore be useful to postgraduates undertaking MRCP, and to medical registrars embarking on a career in cardiology. We hope you enjoy reading.

Acknowledgements

We wish to thank the following for their help: Dr DR Ramsdale, Dr RG Charles, Dr A Harley and Miss K Roebottom (Cardiothoracic Centre, Liverpool), Dr MK Davies (Senior Lecturer in Cardiology, Queen Elizabeth Hospital, Birmingham), Miss S Jones (Senior Chief Physiological Measurement Technician, Queen Elizabeth Hospital) and Miss P Brennan (Chief Physiological Measurement Technician, Birmingham General Hospital). We would also like to thank the Department of Medical Illustration, Selly Oak Hospital, Birmingham, for their help with illustrations.

Case 1

The role of intervention in valvular heart disease

History

A 53-year-old woman gave a 10-year history of increasing shortness of breath on exertion (presently New York Heart Association Class III). She had suffered rheumatic fever as a teenager. On examination the pulse was irregular. The apex beat was tapping and auscultation revealed a loud first heart sound and a quiet mid-diastolic murmur. An electrocardiogram showed atrial fibrillation. An echocardiogram and cardiac catheter study were performed.

Questions

A Describe the echocardiographic appearances (1 and 2).
B What is demonstrated by the catheter findings (3)?
C What can be done to relieve this patient's shortness of breath?

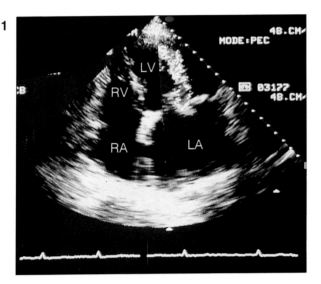

1 Cross-sectional echocardiogram (apical four-chamber view) with colour-flow imaging. LA, left atrium; LV, left ventricle; RA, right atrium; RV, right ventricle.

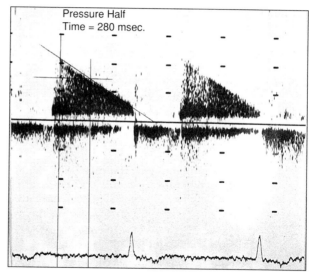

Pressure Half
Time = 280 msec.

2 Continuous wave Doppler
recording of mitral valve flow
obtained from the apex.

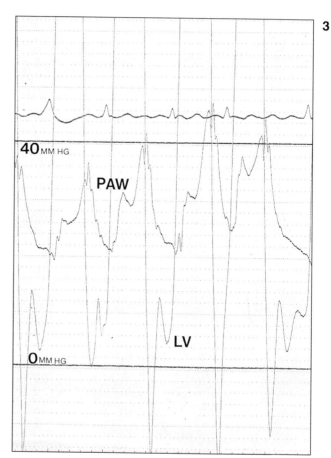

40 MM HG

PAW

LV

0 MM HG

3 Pressures obtained at
catheterization. LV, left
ventricle; PAW, pulmonary
artery wedge. (0–40mmHg
range.)

Case 1

Answers

A A cross-sectional trans-thoracic echocardiogram from the apical four chamber view with colour-flow imaging is shown (1). Colour-flow imaging is essentially a multigate pulsed Doppler technique with information from multiple sample sites. Various colours of variable intensity or mixture are produced representing blood-flow direction, velocity and turbulence. Traditionally, laminar flow towards the transducer is illustrated as red, and laminar flow away from the transducer as blue. This patient shows colour flow 'aliasing' due to high flow velocities in diastole through a stenotic mitral valve. There was no evidence of mitral regurgitation (blue flow into the left atrium in systole) in this case. Continuous wave Doppler is, however, the method of choice for recording velocity waveforms in mitral stenosis. This technique can measure very high velocities, and will not miss the point at which the velocity is greatest, as it measures all velocity changes along the beam. From the desired waveforms (2), several indices can be calculated using the modified Bernoulli equation (peak diastolic gradient, end-diastolic gradient and the pressure half-time). The normal range of the pressure half-time (PHT) for the mitral valve is 20–60ms. This case demonstrates severe obstruction, with a PHT of 280ms and a calculated mitral valve area of 0.8cm^2 (mitral valve area = 220/PHT).

B Cardiac catheterization has traditionally been used to establish the diagnosis and severity of mitral stenosis, although, as described, Doppler can now provide much of this information. The catheter recording (3) shows the pressure gradient across the mitral valve assessed by simultaneous measurement of left atrial pressure obtained indirectly as the pulmonary capillary wedge pressure, and the left ventricular pressure, usually obtained by retrograde catheterization. In mitral stenosis a diastolic pressure gradient occurs which depends on the severity of stenosis and on the flow (in turn, dependent on the cardiac output) across the valve in diastole. In this case the diastolic gradient at rest is considerable (a mean diastolic gradient of 16mmHg and an end-diastolic gradient of 14mmHg). The other important pressure measurement in mitral stenosis is that of pulmonary artery pressure, which in this case was elevated at 50/25mmHg. Further left ventricular angiography showed good left ventricular function with no evidence of mitral regurgitation. Coronary angiography showed normal coronary arteries.

C In view of the severe symptoms and evidence of very significant mitral stenosis, the patient could have been considered for mitral valve replacement or closed mitral commissurotomy. In this case the mitral cusps were stenotic but not calcified, and appeared pliable on echocardiographic examination. To obtain better definition of the mitral valve, trans-oesophageal echocardiography was performed. This confirmed the trans-thoracic findings with thickened and stenotic leaflets. It also showed that the subvalvular apparatus was not involved in the fusion process (4). Furthermore, the left atrium was dilated with spontaneous contrast appearance, but there was no evidence of thrombus formation. In view of such findings percutaneous transluminal mitral commissurotomy (PTMC) was considered feasible and successfully performed using the Inoue balloon catheter. This is a single balloon which is 'flow' directed and steerable across the mitral valve following puncture of the atrial septum. The balloon can be 'anchored' at the stenosed valve during inflation (5–7) and the procedure is usually completed within 1 hour. The mean diastolic gradient was reduced to 2mmHg and the calculated mitral valve area increased to 1.6cm^2, without production of mitral regurgitation. If echocardiography had shown heavy mitral valve calcification and/or subvalvar involvement, mitral valve replacement would be the preferred treatment, as the results of PTMC (like surgical valvotomy) in such cases are often disappointing.

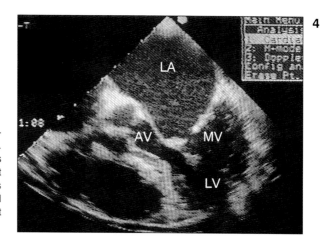

4 Trans-oesophageal echocardiogram showing mitral stenosis. There are thickened mitral leaflets with fused commissures. The left atrium is dilated, with spontaneous contrast appearance. MV, mitral valve; LA, left atrium; LV, left ventricle; AV, aortic valve.

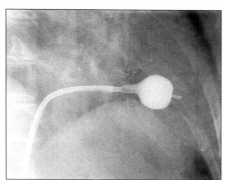

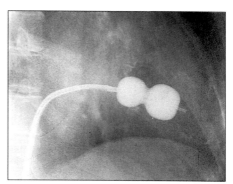

5–7 Sequence of mitral valve dilatation using Inoue's size-adjusting, self-positioning balloon catheter in angiographic right-anterior oblique views. The catheter is floated across the mitral valve into the left ventricle (**5**), where it is partially inflated and then pulled back to anchor the balloon at the mitral valve; (**6**) as the proximal balloon is inflated, a waist is created by the stenosed valve; (**7**) at full inflation, the waist disappears as the commissures are split.

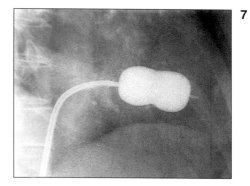

Reference

Inoue K, Hung JS. Percutaneous transvenous mitral commissurotomy (PTMC): The far east experience. In: *Textbook of Interventional Cardiology*. Topol EJ (ed). WB Saunders Co. Ltd, 1990.

Case 2

Severe sepsis in a patient with congenital heart disease

History

A 47-year-old man presented with a four-week history of malaise, lethargy, joint pains, nausea, vomiting and rigors. He had been admitted to a local hospital where he was noted to be pyrexial (39°C). Clinical examination was unremarkable, apart from a pan-systolic murmur on auscultation (the patient was known to have had a small ventricular septal defect since he was a child). In particular, there were no clinical features suggestive of infective endocarditis. Blood cultures grew *Staphylococcus aureus* in all bottles (sensitive to flucloxacillin, fusidic acid or vancomycin). The patient was given flucloxacillin (2g QDS intravenously) for presumed infective endocarditis, but showed no signs of improvement. His fever persisted and he became jaundiced. Investigations showed a progressive rise in white cell count (20.0 × 10^9/l-neutrophilia), fall in haemoglobin (7.9g/dl), thrombocytopenia (platelets 54 000) and hepatocellular jaundice. The ESR was 107mm in 1 hour; C-reactive protein was 219mg/l. An electrocardiogram showed sinus rhythm with a RBBB pattern. The appearance of the chest radiograph is shown in (2). A trans-thoracic echocardiogram was performed and showed a small ventricular septal defect on colour-flow imaging. A trans-oesophageal echocardiogram was then carried out (1).

Questions

A   What does the trans-oesophageal echocardiogram (1) show?
B   What does the chest radiograph (2) show?
C   How would you manage the patient subsequently?

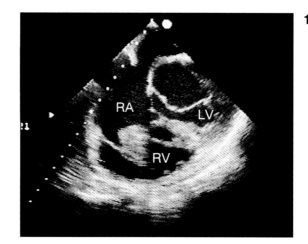

1 Trans-oesophageal echocardiogram. LV, left ventricle; RV, right ventricle; RA, right atrium.

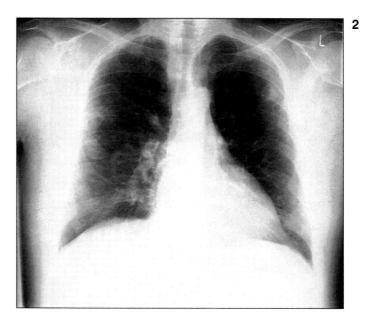

2 Chest radiograph.

Case 2

Answers

A Trans-oesophageal echocardiography (TOE) (1) shows a large vegetation on the posterior leaflet of the tricuspid valve and a smaller vegetation on the anterior leaflet. Vegetations are often difficult to detect by transthoracic echocardiography on right-sided heart lesions, as lesions on the right side of the heart cannot be imaged as well as those on the left. Transoesophageal echocardiography is often very useful, however, in viewing right-sided heart lesions, due to its superior image resolution.

B The chest radiograph(2) shows multiple small cavities in both lung fields which are likely to be lung abscesses. This indicates septic emboli secondary to endocarditis on either a ventricular septal defect (when the left-to-right shunt carries the infected material from the defect into the lungs) or on the tricuspid or pulmonary valves. Abscess formation is frequent if the infecting agent is *Staphylococcus aureus* and the lesions may cavitate. Lung abscesses are particularly common as a complication of the right-sided endocarditis that occurs in intravenous drug abusers because it is usually due to virulent organisms (there was no drug abuse in this case, however).

C This patient has several features indicating the need for surgery in infective endocarditis, namely (i) a large vegetation; (ii) recurrent septic emboli; (iii) signs of infection not resolving on medical therapy (persistent fever, fall in haemoglobin, increasing leucocytosis and deteriorating liver function). In the past, attempts were made to give an adequate course of antibiotics before the operation. Such delay can lead to disastrous results, however, and surgery should be undertaken earlier rather than later in such cases. In this patient the tricuspid valve was excised and the infected vegetations removed. Immediate tricuspid valve replacement with a prosthesis was performed, together with repair of the small ventricular septal defect. The patient was then given a further six weeks of intravenous antibiotics (vancomycin substituted for flucloxacillin).

Reference

Freeman R, Hall RJC. Infective endocarditis. In: *Diseases of the Heart*. Julian DG, Camm AJ, Fox KM, Hall RJC, Poole-Wilson PA (eds). London: Baillière Tindall, 1989.

Problems in a patient with a mechanical prosthetic valve

History

A 54-year-old man presented with a 3-week history of lethargy, aching joints, abdominal pain and diarrhoea. He also had a 3-day history of cough, green sputum and a 'tight' chest. Elective aortic valve replacement 6 years previously (for aortic incompetence associated with a bicuspid valve) had been complicated within one month by infective endocarditis (*Staphylococcus epidermidis*). A further episode of endocarditis 2 years later (culture negative) produced valve dehiscence and required aortic valve re-replacement (Bjork–Shiley prosthesis). The patient had then remained well until this presentation.

On examination a temperature of 37.6°C was noted and the patient looked pale. There were no cutaneous clinical signs suggestive of infective endocarditis. The pulse was 90 beats per minute and regular. Blood pressure was 140/90mmHg. Auscultation revealed satisfactory prosthetic clicks and a soft early diastolic murmur. This murmur had, however, been heard since the second operation and echocardiography had previously shown mild paraprosthetic aortic regurgitation.

A trans-oesophageal echocardiogram (**1**) and an electrocardiogram (**2**) were performed. Haemoglobin was 11g/dl (MCH 28pg; MCHC 32g/dl); white cell count was 11.2 x 10⁹/l. Chest radiograph was normal apart from mild cardiomegaly. C-reactive protein was 102mg/l. Urinalysis was negative. All blood cultures were sterile. Trans-thoracic and trans-oesophageal echocardiograms were performed.

Questions

A What is the likely cause of the patient's present symptoms?
B What does the trans-oesophageal echocardiogram (**1**) show?
C Comment on the patient's further management.

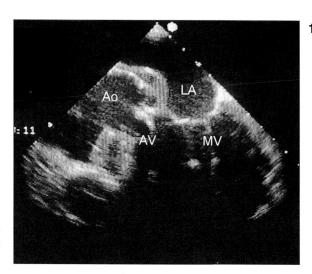

1 Trans-oesophageal echocardiogram. LA, left atrium; Ao, aorta; AV, aortic valve; MV, mitral valve.

Case 3

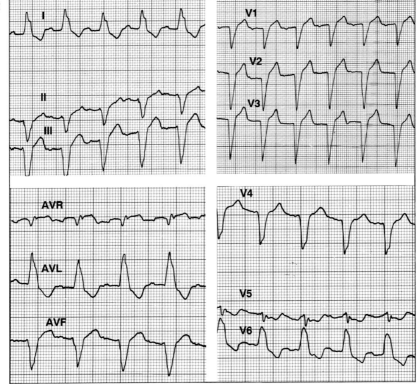

2 12-lead electrocardiogram at admission.

Answers

A A diagnosis of recurrent prosthetic valve endocarditis requires a high index of suspicion in this case, and should be suspected in any patient with a prosthetic valve who has unexplained fever, generalized ill-health or a new murmur. Mortality is extremely high (ranging from 30–50%) and all patients should be managed in a centre where cardiac surgery is available. In patients with mechanical prostheses, infection always involves the paravalvular tissues, thereby undermining attachment of the valve and often leading to necrosis with abscess formation. The most important findings in this case are the electro-cardiographic abnormalities (2) of left bundle branch block (noted on previous electro-cardiograms) and first degree heart block (a new finding), suggesting the possibility of intra-myocardial spread of the infection with abscess formation near the conducting tissue.

B Trans-thoracic echocardiography (TTE) showed nothing abnormal apart from mild aortic incompetence. TTE, however, often fails to identify vegetations on prosthetic valves, as strong reflections from the prosthetic valve tend to overshadow the more delicate reflections from the vegetations. The detection of vegetations and abscess formation is improved considerably using trans-oesophageal echocardiography. Imaging is done in the near field of the echotransducer and resolution is much higher. In this case it clearly shows an aortic root abscess (discrete echo-free space between the aorta and left atrium) but no vegetations were seen (1).

C Emergency surgery is required in such cases. In this case, examination of the prosthetic valve at operation showed dehiscence for more than 50% of its circumference (due to infection with associated root abscesses). An abscess at the commissure extended into the right ventricle as a fistula. The valve was excised and the abscesses extensively debrided. The aortic-right ventricular fistula was repaired using a patch of pericardium. A 25mm homograft aortic root was inserted and the left/right coronary arteries were reimplanted into the homograft. The patient had an uneventful post-operative recovery. He was given intravenous benzyl penicillin for 6 weeks, together with gentamycin for the first 2 weeks. The patient remained in complete heart block and, therefore, a dual chamber permanent pacing system was inserted.

Reference

Freeman R, Hall RJC. Infective endocarditis. In: *Diseases of the Heart.* Julian DG, Camm AJ, Fox KM, Hall RJC, Poole-Wilson PA (eds). London: Baillière Tindall, 1989.

Case 4

Severe heart failure in a young man

History

A 25-year-old man presented with hypotension, tachycardia, painless jaundice, and a week-long non-specific 'flu like' illness with sore throat and nasal stuffiness prior to presentation. His job involved the retail of paints and wallpaper. One month prior to the illness he had been immersed in a local stream. Jaudice with dark urine had developed on the day of admission. During the admission he developed acute renal failure requiring emergency peritoneal dialysis. A renal biopsy subsequently revealed acute tubular necrosis. He became increasingly hypotensive despite inotropic support. An echocardiogram showed severe dilatation of both ventricles with a calculated left ventricular ejection fraction of <10%. There was mitral and tricuspid incompetence but these lesions were assumed to be functional. No valvar vegetations were identified. Cardiac catheterization revealed pulmonary artery pressure 50/28mmHg, left ventricular pressure 80/12–26mmHg, and aortic pressure 80/52mmHg. Selective coronary arterography revealed normal coronary arteries. A left ventricular biopsy was performed (1). After a period of intensive support there was a complete recovery of cardiac and renal function. During recovery the left ventricular biopsy was repeated (2).

Questions

A What does the biopsy (1) show?
B What aetiological agents could be responsible for these changes?

1
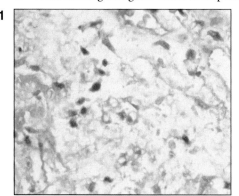
2
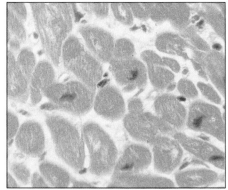

1 Left ventricular endomyocardial biopsy.

2 Repeated left ventricular biopsy after clinical recovery.

Answers

A The left ventricular biopsy shows severe haemorrhagic myocarditis.
B Infective causes such as leptospirosis, viral myocarditis and Han-Tan virus, and occupational causes such as exposure to organic solvents should all be considered. Subsequent serology for leptospirosis, blood cultures and viral titres were all negative in this case, and no cause has been identified for the episode of acute haemorrhagic myocarditis in this patient. Repeat biopsy after clinical recovery showed normal histological appearance (2).

Syncope before and after permanent pacemaker implantation

History

A 78-year-old woman with a recent history of recurrent syncope and dizziness was referred to a cardiologist. Clinical examination was unremarkable. An electrocardiogram showed sinus rhythm with first degree atrioventricular block. A 24 hour Holter recording showed sinus bradycardia (minimum heart rate 28 beats per minute at 11.00 hours) and intermittent 2:1 atrioventricular block. A permanent pacemaker system using a ventricular demand pacemaker (VVI) was implanted. The patient re-presented to the casualty department the following week with further episodes of dizziness and syncope. She was now noted to be hypotensive (blood pressure supine 100/70mmHg; blood pressure standing 85/60mmHg). The casualty officer reported satisfactory pacemaker function following an electrocardiogram (1).

Questions

A What does the electrocardiogram (1) show?
B What condition has the patient re-presented with?
C How would you manage the patient subsequently?

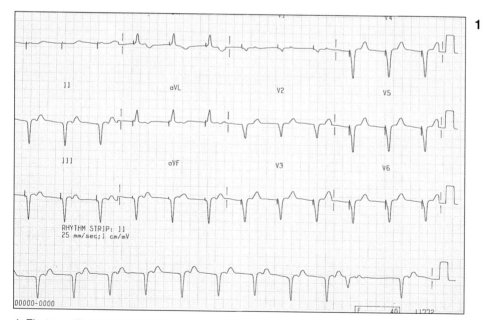

1 Electrocardiogram at presentation to casualty department.

Case 5

Answers

A The electrocardiogram (1) shows single-chamber ventricular demand pacing with a VVI pacemaker. When discussing pacemakers, it is helpful to be familiar with the three-letter code used to describe the various pacing modes available. The first letter of the code refers to the chamber that is paced (A = atrium, V = ventricle, and D = both atrium and ventricle). The second letter refers to the chamber that is sensed (again, A, V, or D; in addition, the letter O is used if there is no sensing). The third letter refers to the mode of response when an event is sensed (I = inhibited, T = triggered, D = either inhibited or triggered, depending on circumstances, O = neither inhibited or triggered). In other words VVI pacemakers pace the ventricle at a fixed rate (in this patient at 70 per minute) whenever the intrinsic ventricular rate falls below that fixed rate. Any intrinsic rhythm within the pacemaker escape interval (e.g a ventricular extrasystole in this case) is sensed, the pacemaker is inhibited from firing and the escape interval subsequently reset.

More careful inspection of the electrocardiogram in this patient shows that each paced complex is immediately followed by a p wave due to retrograde atrial activation (i.e. impulses originating in the ventricles are transmitted backward to the atria). In this situation, each ventricular paced beat is virtually guaranteed to produce an atrial contraction during ventricular systole.

B The patient has re-presented with 'pacemaker syndrome'. Normal atrioventricular synchronization is lost in VVI pacing and atrial contraction may occur against closed mitral and tricuspid valves. The loss of properly timed atrial systole results in a reduction in cardiac output of up to one-third and may cause hypotension; near-syncope and syncope can result. Ventriculo-atrial conduction, as seen in this case, causes even greater haemodynamic upset, and the resultant atrial distension may actually initiate a reflex vasodepressor effect. The hypotension is often more marked whilst standing, as seen in this case.

C Ventricular pacing is unsuitable for patients who are mainly in sinus rhythm but who often develop bradycardia at a rate less than the cycle length of the ventricular pacemaker, i.e. those with sick sinus or carotid sinus syndromes. Reprogramming the pacemaker rate to a value below the intrinsic sinus rate (2) abolishes the problem but left this patient with symptomatic sinus bradycardia and a junctional escape rhythm. The patient's pacemaker system was therefore 'upgraded' with an atrial lead and a dual-chamber (DDD) pacemaker (using the original ventricular lead) to produce atrioventricular sequential pacing (3). This prevented further episodes of hypotension and syncope.

Reference

Serge Barold S. *Modern cardiac pacing.* New York: Futura, 1985.

2

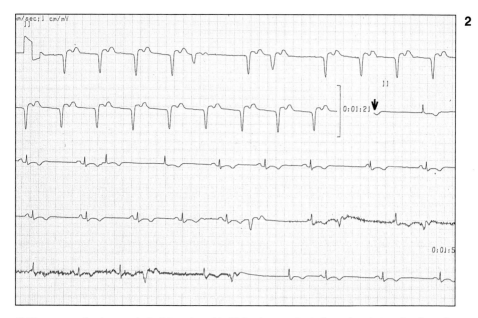

2 The pacemaker lower rate limit is reduced to 30 beats per minute (arrow) and sinus bradycardia returns.

3

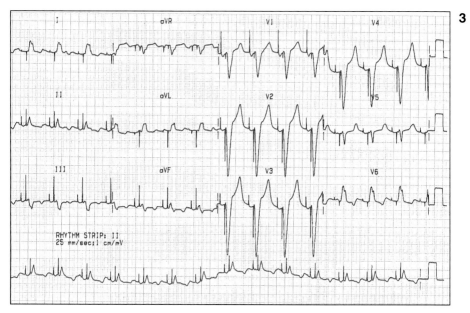

3 Physiological pacing (DDD pacemaker) showing atrial and ventricular pacing (i.e. maintenance of A-V synchrony).

A 'syndrome' with cardiac malformations

History

A 48-year-old man presented to a cardiology clinic with a 12-month history of shortness of breath on exertion, and palpitations. Clinical examination revealed short stature and an unusual clinical appearance. The pulse was irregular. Palpation of the precordium revealed an active cardiac impulse of right ventricular type. Auscultation revealed a split second heart sound and an ejection systolic murmur heard at the upper left sternal edge. An electrocardiogram showed atrial fibrillation and a right bundle branch block pattern.

Questions

A What 'syndrome' does the physical appearance (1 and 2) suggest?
B What does the patient's chest radiograph (3) show?
C What does the patient's cross-sectional echocardiogram (4) show?
D What further investigations are required in this patient?

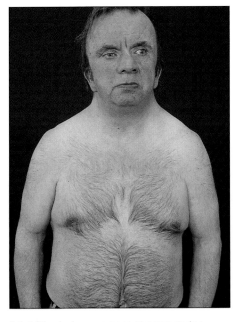
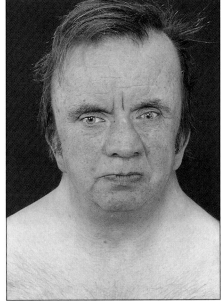

1 & 2 Physical appearance at presentation.

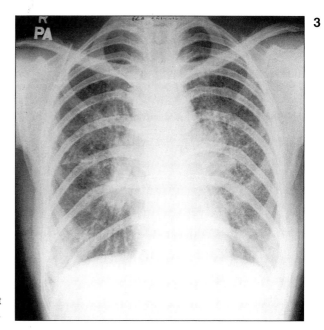

3 Chest radiograph at presentation.

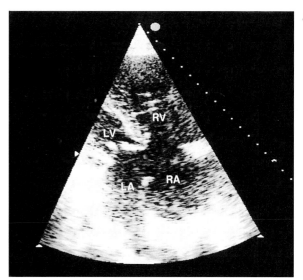

4 Cross-sectional echocardiogram (apical four-chamber view). RA, right atrium; LA, left atrium; RV, right ventricle; LV, left ventricle.

Case 6

Answers

A The striking abnormalities in the patient's physical appearance – short webbed neck, low-set ears, short stature – are characteristic of 'Noonan's' syndrome. This syndrome has an autosomal dominant mode of inheritance. Such patients are often retarded (although not in this case) and exhibit down-slanting palpebral fissures, cryptorchidism and pectus excavatum/carinatum. The cardiac abnormalities associated with this syndrome are pulmonary valve stenosis, atrial septal defect and hypertrophic cardiomyopathy.

B The chest radiograph (3) shows that the pulmonary trunk is very prominent and the normal peripheral vascular pattern is accentuated. These features are consistent with conditions causing an increase in pulmonary blood flow.

C The cross-sectional echocardiogram (4) is an apical four-chamber view, which in this case demonstrates a primum atrial septal defect. Cross-sectional echocardiography has revolutionized the diagnosis of such defects. The four-chamber views are the most useful, from either apical or subcostal windows, particularly when used in combination with contrast echocardiograhy, pulsed Doppler or colour-flow mapping. Enlargement of the right ventricle and right atrium is also seen here.

D Cardiac catheterization is usually deemed necessary in such cases to quantify the severity of intracardiac shunt. A left-to-right shunt is usually detected at atrial level by a rise in oxygen saturation. Subsequent rises in oxygen saturation in the right ventricle or pulmonary trunk may also occur if there is an associated atrioventricular canal malformation. At catheterization, the left atrium is easily entered in the majority of patients. Most important, however, is the presence or absence of pulmonary hypertension. In this case only a shunt at atrial level was demonstrated and the pulmonary artery pressure was normal. The left-to-right shunt was quantified as 2.5:1 and surgical repair was, therefore, recommended. The patient was also anticoagulated to prevent potential thromboembolism associated with atrial fibrillation.

Reference

Duncan WJ, Fowler RS, Farkas LG, *et al.* A comprehensive scoring system for evaluating Noonan's syndrome. *Am J Med Genet* 1981; **10**:37-50.

Collapse associated with raised intra-thoracic pressure

History

A 38-year-old woman collapsed suddenly whilst straining on the toilet. There was no relevant medical history and she had been feeling perfectly well until the episode of collapse. On admission to hospital she complained of anterior chest discomfort and dyspnoea. Examination revealed evidence of tachycardia and hypotension, and there was a long early diastolic murmur audible over the sternal edge. Echocardiography was performed.

Questions

A What diagnoses would you consider in this case?
B What do the echocardiographic appearances (1) and (2) show?

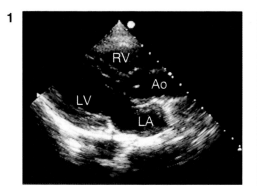 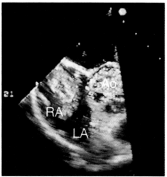

1 Trans-thoracic echocardiogram (parasternal long-axis view). RV, right ventricle; LV, left ventricle; LA, left atrium; Ao, aorta.

2 Trans-oesophageal echocardiogram with colour flow Doppler. RA, right atrium; LA, left atrium; Ao, aorta.

Answers

A The most likely diagnosis would be an acute pulmonary embolus. However, in this case it would not have accounted for the diastolic murmur, and a perfusion/ventilation isotope scan was negative. A 12-lead electrocardiogram revealed non-specific ST/T wave changes in the lateral leads and a chest X-ray showed minor cardiomegaly only.

B A trans-thoracic echocardiogram (1) revealed dilation of the aortic root and prominence of the sinus of Valsalva. A trans-oesophageal echocardiogram later revealed evidence of a ruptured sinus of Valsalva aneurysm with the development of an aortic-right atrial fistula (2).

Case 8

Heart failure with good ventricular contractility

History

A 60-year-old man was referred to the cardiology unit from a local district general hospital. He had been admitted with progressive dyspnoea, ankle swelling, loss of previous stamina and fatigue. He also complained of a long-standing cough with productive sputum. He was previously a heavy cigarette smoker. He had been treated for tuberculosis twenty years previously. On examination, a raised jugular venous pressure was noted, together with hepatomegaly, ascites and marked peripheral oedema. Auscultation revealed a third heart sound but no murmurs. An electrocardiogram showed sinus rhythm with inverted T waves in the precordial leads. The chest radiograph is shown in (1) and (2). The patient was diagnosed as having cor pulmonale secondary to chronic lung disease and was treated with bronchodilators and diuretics. His condition did not improve and a progressive rise in blood urea and creatinine was noted. The blood pressure decreased and the patient became oliguric. An echocardiogram was performed which showed normal sized cardiac chambers and good left ventricular function. The patient later underwent cardiac catheter studies at the regional cardiac unit (3 and 4) after his clinical condition had improved.

Questions

A   What condition does this patient suffer from?
B   What other investigations would have proved useful?
C   What do the catheter pressure tracings show?
D   Why did the patient's renal function deteriorate?
E   What further treatment should be recommended in this case?

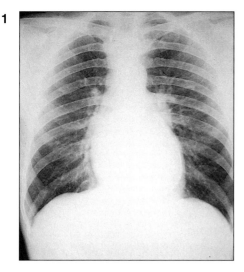

1 Chest radiograph (P-A view).

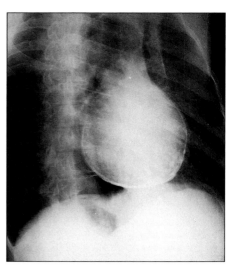

2 Right lateral chest radiograph.

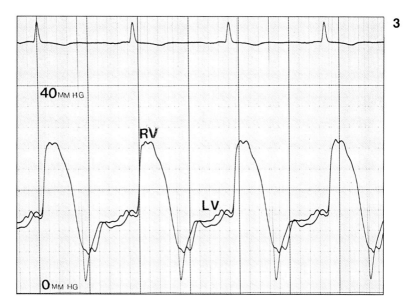

3 Simultaneous recording of left (LV) and right (RV) ventricular pressure (0–40mmHg range).

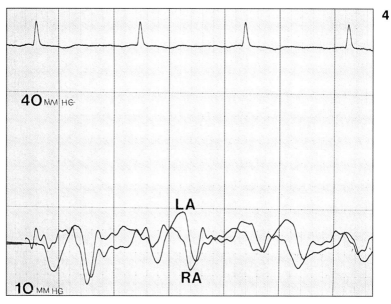

4 Simultaneous right atrial (RA) and left atrial (LA) pressure recordings (10–40mmHg range).

Case 8

Answers

A Careful viewing of the chest radiograph shows a rim of calcium encasing the heart, suggesting a diagnosis of calcific constrictive pericarditis. This is best seen on penetrated postero-anterior (P-A) views and on the lateral (2). The history and physical signs also suggest this diagnosis. The third heart sound, in this case, is a pericardial knock due to early abrupt cessation of rapid diastolic filling of the ventricles. Tuberculosis is the most likely cause of constrictive pericarditis in this instance, although it is not the most common cause seen today. Many cases nowadays are not associated with any preceding illness, and the pericardium is not necessarily calcified. It should also be remembered that calcification of the pericardium may be seen with similar distribution in patients with no evidence of constriction.

B Echocardiography does not show pericardial thickening in most cases of constriction and is, therefore, not a diagnostic investigation in this condition. The fact that it demonstrated good left ventricular function in this case, however, was helpful. Computed tomography is a very useful investigation for non-invasive recognition of pericardial thickening. This is usually clearly visible, with a high-density line of thickening around the heart that contrasts with the inner low-density epicardial fat layer (5).

C Cardiac catheterization is often unnecessary in typical cases of constrictive pericarditis, although, along with computed tomography, it is required to differentiate this condition from restrictive cardiomyopathy in difficult cases. (3) and (4) show typical pressure tracings in constriction. They reveal similarity of the diastolic pressure in all four chambers to within a millimetre or two. The right ventricular diastolic pressure is high in constriction (unless the patient has undergone excessive diuresis). The shape of the diastolic pressure in the left and right ventricles (3) produces the well known 'square root' sign, with a low early diastolic pressure (rapid early filling) and rapid rise to a plateau during diastasis. Also note the prominent 'y' descent (4), indicating that atrial emptying is rapid and unimpeded in early diastole.

D The patient received increasing diuretics for presumed right heart failure, which produced hypovolaemia with hypotension and pre-renal failure. This was treated successfully with cautious intravenous rehydration.

E Pericardiectomy, involving removal of the pericardium from the surface of both ventricles, is recommended. In advanced cases, however, there is a high risk of operative mortality. In this patient the visceral pericardium was involved, with no clear plane of dissection. This made the operation difficult and tedious but the outcome was successful.

Reference

Cameron J, Oesterle SN, Baldwin JC, *et al.* The aetiologic spectrum of constricted pericarditis. *Am Heart J* 1987; **113**: 354-360.

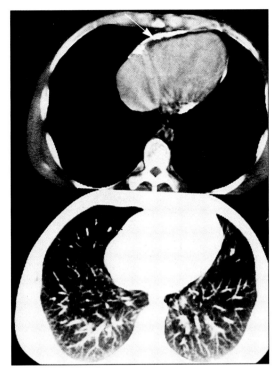

5 Computed tomograms of (top) the thorax, showing dense and thickened pericardium (arrow), and (bottom) the abdomen, showing dilated hepatic veins.

Embolic events in a young patient

History

A 38-year-old woman presented with sudden loss of vision in her right eye associated with left arm and leg weakness. The patient was previously well, apart from occasional palpitations. She was a life-long non-smoker and was on no medication. Clinical examination revealed complete visual loss in the right eye and the fundal appearance is shown in (1). Cardiovascular examination revealed an irregular pulse and a systolic murmur, heard at the apex. No carotid bruits were heard. The patient regained full power in her limbs within six hours, but the visual defect remained static. An initial electrocardiogram showed atrial fibrillation which reverted spontaneously to sinus rhythm the same day. Two echocardiograms (2 and 3) and a phonocardiogram (4) were performed.

Questions

A   What fundal changes are shown in (1)?
B   What are the echocardiographic findings in (2) and (3)?
C   What does the phonocardiogram (4) show?
D   What investigations should be performed?
E   What further treatment would you advise for this patient?

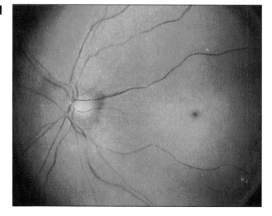

1 Fundal appearance at presentation.

Case 9

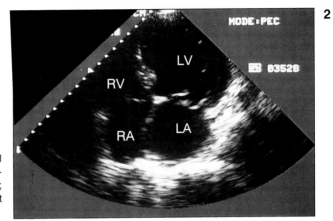

2 Trans-thoracic cross-sectional echocardiogram (apical four-chamber view). LV, left ventricle; RV, right ventricle; LA, left atrium; RA, right atrium.

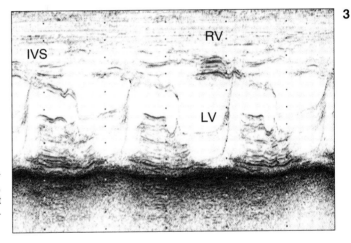

3 M-mode echocardiogram appearance. RV, right ventricle; LV, left ventricle; IVS, interventricular septum.

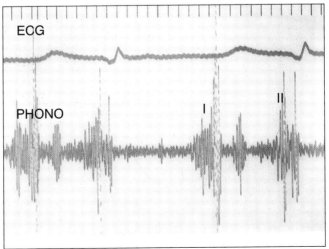

4 Simultaneous (100mm/s) electrocardiogram (ECG) and phonocardiogram (PHONO).

29

29

Case 9

Answers

A This is a classic fundal picture of central retinal artery occlusion, the arteries being transformed into narrow threads. The whole fundus appears pale and there is a 'cherry-red' spot at the macula (red choroid showing through this thin area of retina). Optic atrophy developed later in this case.

B The cross-sectional echocardiogram (2) clearly shows the posterior cusp of the mitral valve protruding back into the left atrium (the recording was taken in late systole). The M-mode echocardiogram (3) reveals pan-systolic 'hammocking' of the posterior cusp of the mitral valve. Furthermore, the excursion of the anterior cusp of the mitral valve is wide, coming into contact with the interventricular septum (a non-specific finding in mitral prolapse). Mild mitral regurgitation (not shown) was demonstrated by Doppler echocardiography.

C The phonocardiogram (4), recorded from the apex, reveals a mid-systolic click followed by a systolic murmur which is present up to the second heart sound (II): classic findings of mitral valve prolapse. The first heart sound is also shown (I).

D The patient presented with a serious embolic event associated with mitral valve prolapse. Both stroke and transient ischaemic attacks are more prevalent in this condition. Emboli originating at areas of endothelial damage on the atrial surface of the valve, caused by the valve's abnormal structure and mobility, have been postulated as the cause. The onset of atrial fibrillation may also have contributed to the embolic event, and atrial and ventricular arrhythmias are probably more common in mitral prolapse than the normal population. Ambulatory Holter monitoring for arrhythmias is therefore an appropriate investigation in this patient. It is also important to exclude infective endocarditis as a potential source of emboli in this situation, and in this case the result was indeed negative.

E The patient should receive full anticoagulation with heparin followed by warfarin, although the benefit over antiplatelet agents (aspirin, dipyridamole) in such cases is unknown. No antiarrhythmic prophylaxis to prevent recurrent atrial fibrillation (e.g. flecainide, propafenone) was initiated, although it would have to be considered if further arrhythmias occurred.

Reference

Barnett HJM, Boughner DR, Taylor DW, *et al.* Further evidence relating mitral valve prolapse to cerebral ischaemic events. *N Engl J Med* 1980; **302**:139-144.

Endocarditis with an unusual echocardiogram appearance

History

A 28-year-old man presented at a haematology clinic with fever and malaise, after his general practitioner had found evidence of microcytic anaemia on a blood count. Three months previously he had had routine dental treatment which included scaling. Blood culture identified *Streptococcus sanguis* in all three culture bottles. An echocardiogram showed a possible vegetation on the aortic valve which was thought to be bicuspid. A trans-oesophageal echocardiogram was performed (1) which confirmed the appearance of an aortic valve vegetation, and in addition a prominence of the aortic wall at the aorto-mitral continuity.

Question

A How has the trans-oesophageal echocardiogram (1) contributed to the management of this patient?

1

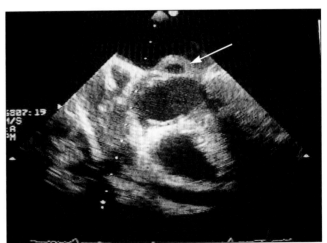

1 Trans-oesophageal echocardiogram appearance in the region of the aortic root.

Answer

A The trans-oesophageal echocardiogram (1) confirmed vegetations associated with the aortic valve leaflets and demonstrated an aneurysmal dilatation of the aorto-mitral continuity (arrow) that was not seen on the trans-thoracic study. This area is commonly affected by abscess formation and/or aneurysmal dilatation in aortic valve endocarditis. Both abnormalities are difficult to discern via conventional echocardiography. The aneurysmal dilatation occurs in an area of turbulence at the aorto-mitral annulus and can enlarge progressively, with risk of rupture or fistula formation.

Case 11

Cardiovascular manifestations of a systemic disease

History

A 28-year-old woman presented with a 2-day history of severe shortness of breath with cough. There were no other symptoms. She had previously experienced two episodes of spontaneous pneumothorax. She also admitted to bruising very easily and said other family members were similarly affected. On examination, there was an increased respiratory rate. The pulse was 120 beats/min, regular and of small volume. Blood pressure was 110/60mmHg. The apex beat was displaced laterally and was heaving in character. Auscultation revealed a gallop rhythm, a systolic and short diastolic murmur and crepitations at the lung bases. An electrocardiogram showed left ventricular hypertrophy with prominent Q waves in the antero-lateral leads. A chest radiograph revealed cardiomegaly and pulmonary venous congestion. Echocardiography was performed and the results are shown in (1) and (2).

Questions

A What do the echocardiograms (1 and 2) show and what are the auscultatory findings due to?

B The clinical appearance of this patient's skin is shown in (3). What abnormalities are seen, what other features may be present and what cardiovascular complications may occur in this condition?

C What further investigations are required in this patient?

D What treatment should this patient receive?

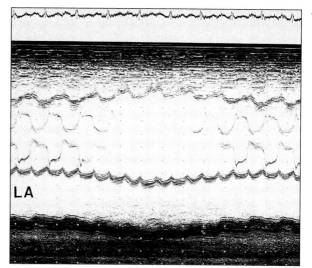

1 M-mode echocardiogram. LA, left atrium.

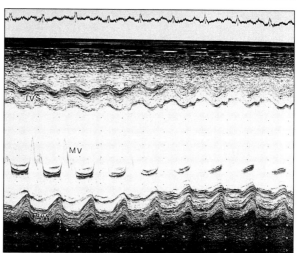

2 M-mode echocardiogram. IVS, interventricular septum; PVW, posterior ventricular wall; MV, mitral valve.

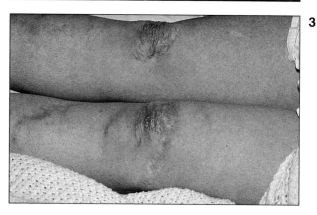

3 Skin appearance.

Case 11

Answers

A The M-mode echocardiogram (parasternal long-axis view) in (1) shows an enormously dilated aortic root measuring 5.5cm at the level of the aortic valve and increasing to 6.5cm as the ultrasonic beam scans superiorly (the upper limit of normal for the aortic dimension is 4cm, measured in diastole, i.e. the R wave on the electrocardiogram). This condition is known as 'aortic annulus ectasia', which leads to a central defect whereby the three aortic cusps fail to meet and hence aortic regurgitation occurs (confirmed by Doppler examination).

The M-mode echocardiogram of the left ventricle (parasternal long-axis view) in (2) shows marked dilatation of the left ventricle (diastolic diameter 8cm [normal up to 5.5cm]; systolic diameter 6.5cm [normal up to 4cm]). Marked impairment of contractility of the interventricular septum and posterior ventricular wall is also visible. Note that the mitral valve closes well before the onset of the next QRS complex, despite a fast heart rate. This is due to an early rise in left ventricular diastolic pressure (caused by torrential regurgitation). These findings indicate a background of chronic severe aortic regurgitation. The short history suggests an acute event, however, and in this case it is likely that acute regurgitation has occurred in someone who already has a significant degree of chronic aortic regurgitation. This leads to a mixed clinical picture with some signs of chronic regurgitation but with tachycardia, pulmonary oedema and heart failure. The latter produces a gallop rhythm, shortening of the early diastolic murmur and a decrease in pulse pressure. A pansystolic murmur is also sometimes present at the cardiac apex in advanced cases in whom left ventricular dilatation leads to functional mitral regurgitation.

B (3) shows fragile atrophic skin (a senile appearance called acrogeria) which has healed poorly (and bruises easily). This is characteristic of Ehlers–Danlos (ED) syndrome, a term that applies to a group of diseases (of at least 10 types) which are extremely rare and usually inherited by well-defined dominant or recessive traits. Hyperextensibility of the joints due to lax ligaments is an associated feature. Some groups have a tendency to other manifestations including kyphoscoliosis, intestinal rupture and spontaneous pneumothorax. The cardiac features are similar to those of Marfan's syndrome, with cystic medial necrosis leading to aortic root dilatation (as in this case) and aortic dissection with minimal trauma, especially secondary to arterial catheterization. Spontaneous rupture and dissection of other arteries can also occur. Floppy mitral valve and abnormal atrioventricular conduction are other manifestations.

C As vascular rupture can easily occur during cardiac catheterization in patients with ED syndrome, it should be carried out only if there is insufficient information from non-invasive investigations. In this case the extent of aortic root involvement required evaluation prior to cardiac surgery and aortography was therefore performed (4). It is usually impossible to obtain coronary angiography in this situation and extreme care should be taken during aortography, particularly if there is any question of aortic dissection. Trans-oesophageal echocardiography may nowadays be a more appropriate investigation in such circumstances (5).

D There is no specific treatment for ED syndrome. In this particular case the aortic root was excised and replaced with a homograft. The coronary arteries were reimplanted into the homograft and the patient made a full recovery.

Reference

Madison WM, Bradley E, Castilo A. Ehlers–Danlos syndrome with cardiac involvement. *Am J Cardiol* 1963; **11**:689-693.

Case 11

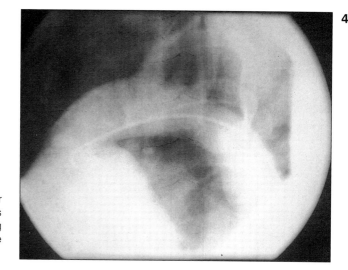

4 Supraventricular aortogram showing gross dilatation of the ascending aorta, with sparing of the great vessels.

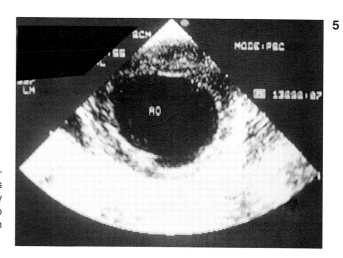

5 Trans-oesophageal echo-cardiogram in aortic annulus ectasia showing a massively dilated aortic root. No dissection was present in this case. Ao, Aorta.

The histology of unstable angina

History

A 47-year-old man was admitted to a coronary care unit with a 24-hour history of chest pain at rest associated with symmetrical T wave inversion in the anterior-septal leads. Serial creatinine phosphokinase levels were measured and found to be within the normal range. Treatment with aspirin, beta-adrenoreceptor blockade and intravenous nitrates was instituted, with a prompt clinical response. Left heart catheterization and coronary angiography were performed on the second hospital day. The study demonstrated normal left ventricular contraction with a severe sub-total eccentric stenosis of the left anterior descending (LAD) artery, before the origin of the first septal branch (1). Directional coronary atherectomy (DCA) was performed as an interval procedure 3 weeks after the resolution of chest pain on the ground of the higher risk associated with coronary interventional procedures in the early phase of unstable angina. The procedure is outlined in (2) to (4). There was a good angiographic result and the procedure was uncomplicated. The patient remained free of angina at follow up. The histology of the atheromatous material is shown in (5). Evidence of plaque stabilization by neo-vascularization was seen within 3 weeks of the onset of chest pain. These appearances may explain the clinical resolution of this episode of unstable angina.

Question

A What was the likely cause of this episode of unstable angina?

1

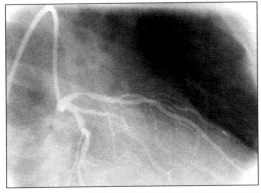

1 Left coronary angiogram (posterior-anterior projection). Severe subtotal occlusion is seen in the left anterior descending artery (arrow).

2

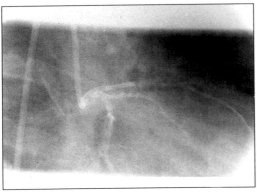

2 Outline of procedure of DCA.

3

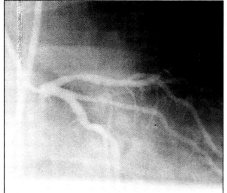

4

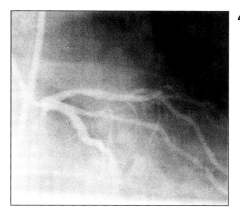

3 & 4 Outline of procedure of DCA.

5

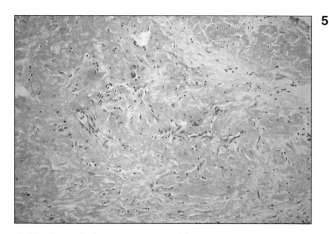

5 Histology of atheromatous material.

Answer

A The mechanism now considered most likely for the development of 'acute coronary syndromes' (infarction or unstable angina) is the rupture of a pre-existing atheromatous plaque. This exposes sub-endothelial components of the plaque that cause an adherent secondary thrombus. The thrombotic element appears to be responsible for the high complication rate in early angioplasty of acute coronary occlusion. Stabilization of the plaque by neo-vascularization, as seen in this case, may account for the resolution of symptoms that occurs with medical therapy in the majority of patients with unstable angina.

Reference

Myler RK, Shaw RE *et al.* Unstable angina and coronary angioplasty. *Circulation* 1990; 82(2):88-95.

Case 13

An unusual cause of right heart failure

History

A 59-year-old man presented with a 6-month history of increasing tiredness, reduced effort tolerance, ankle swelling, abdominal discomfort and diarrhoea. He also noticed a feeling of uncomfortable fullness in the neck and face from time to time. There was no medical history of note. Cardiovascular examination revealed that the jugular venous pressure was elevated. Auscultation revealed a soft systolic murmur and a moderate diastolic murmur, both heard at the apex and left sternal edge. The liver was enlarged and ascites were present, together with moderate ankle oedema. An echocardiogram (1) and Doppler examination (2) were performed and cardiac catheter studies were subsequently carried out (3). His facial appearance is shown in (4).

Questions

A   What does the echocardiogram (1) show?
B   What does the Doppler examination (2) show?
C   What does the cardiac catheter recording (3) show?
D   What is the likely diagnosis and what further investigations are required?
E   How would you treat this condition?

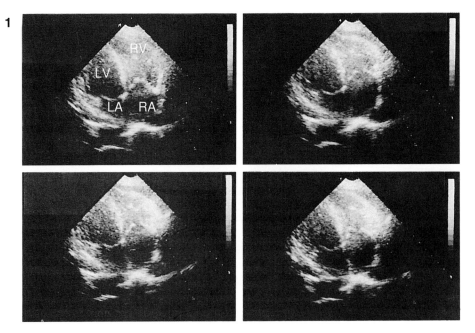

1 Cross-sectional echocardiogram in four-chamber view (right ventricle on right of each frame). RV, right ventricle; RA, right atrium; LV, left ventricle; LA, left atrium.

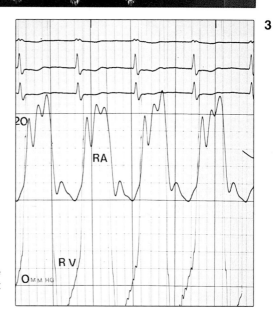

2 Continuous wave Doppler recording (right ventricle now on left of frame image).

3 Simultaneous measurement of pressure in the right atrium (RA) and the right ventricle (RV). (0–20mmHg range.)

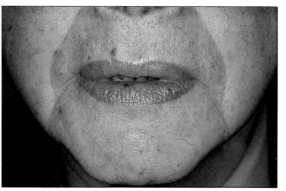

4 Facial appearance.

Case 13

Answers

A The cross-sectional echocardiogram (**1**) shows enlargement of the right ventricle and right atrium compared to the left chambers. The tricuspid leaflets are irregularly thickened and have a high reflectance compared to the mitral valve. In this case the tricuspid valve was fixed in a semi-open position throughout the cardiac cycle.

B The continuous wave Doppler tracing recorded across the tricuspid valve (**2**) shows a significant diastolic gradient (increased peak velocity and slow rate of decline of velocity) together with a significant regurgitant jet between the right ventricle and right atrium during systole (velocity of approximately 3.5m/s). No mitral diastolic gradient or regurgitation was demonstrated by Doppler examination, however.

C The catheter recording (**3**) shows simultaneous pressure measurements (by two separate catheters) from the right atrium and right ventricle. This reveals an end-diastolic pressure difference across the tricuspid valve of 10mmHg, together with features consistent with tricuspid regurgitation (prominent 'V' wave and a sharp 'y' descent). The right ventricular end-diastolic pressure is normal, however.

D The echocardiographic, Doppler and cardiac catheter findings suggest very significant tricuspid stenosis and regurgitation. The symptoms and physical signs of right heart failure are consistent with this diagnosis. Tricuspid stenosis is nearly always rheumatic in origin but in this case there was no history of rheumatic fever and both the mitral and aortic valves appeared structurally normal. Other causes of tricuspid stenosis are exceedingly rare, including sarcoma or a secondary deposit from a tumour. In this case there is a mixture of stenosis and regurgitation, and echocardiography shows that the tricuspid valve is fixed in a mid position through the cardiac cycle. This fact, the presence of telangiectasia and history of facial fullness (flushing was not present) indicate the possibility of a diagnosis of carcinoid syndrome.

The diagnosis of carcinoid syndrome is usually made from a history (humoral consequences of neoplastic enterochromaffin cells) of cutaneous flushing, diarrhoea, bronchoconstriction, valvar lesions on the right side of the heart (tricuspid and/or pulmonary) and facial telangiectasia (**4**). It is confirmed by an elevated 24-hour excretion of 5-hydroxyindole acetic acid (5HIAA) in the urine. Liver ultrasonography may demonstrate tumour deposits, while liver biopsy may produce a positive tissue diagnosis. A marked increase in the urinary output of 5HIAA was observed in this case and hepatic tumour deposits were confirmed on biopsy.

E Patients with carcinoid syndrome need regular careful assessment and treatment of new problems. Cyproheptadine is a specific 5-HT antagonist which may be helpful in controlling diarrhoea and flushing, while somatostatin analogues may also be useful. The prognosis is variable (some patients survive 20 years or more) but cardiac involvement is a common cause of death. Apart from symptomatic cardiac treatment, valve replacement (and, recently, reports of balloon valvuloplasty) has an important role in alleviating symptoms.

References

Littler WA. Carcinoid heart disease. In: *Diseases of the heart.* Julian DG, Camm AJ, Fox KM, Hall RJC, Poole-Wilson PA (eds). London: Baillière Tindall, 1989.

Wilde P. *Doppler echocardiography – An illustrated clinical guide.* London: Churchill Livingstone, 1989.

An unusual cause of haemoptysis

History

A 60-year-old man with long-standing exertional dyspnoea presented with sudden haemoptysis. On examination finger clubbing was noted. Cardiovascular and respiratory examination was normal. An electrocardiogram and chest radiograph were also reported as normal, as was a bronchoscopy. A diagnosis of pulmonary embolism was suggested and the patient was treated with intravenous heparin pending a ventilation-perfusion isotope lung scan. Further severe haemoptysis occurred and an emergency pulmonary angiogram was performed (1).

Questions

A What is the correct diagnosis in this case?
B What associated syndrome may this patient have?
C What other investigations may prove useful in this patient?
D What complications can occur in this condition?
E What treatment can this patient be offered?

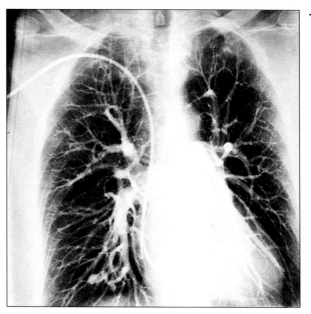

1 Pulmonary angiogram appearance.

Case 14

Answers

A The pulmonary angiogram (1) shows an arteriovenous fistula or malformation in the right lower lobe. Such fistulas can be multiple and result from an abnormality of capillary development in the lungs. Generally, they have a single feeding artery, which is a branch of the pulmonary artery, and drain into a pulmonary vein. The classic clinical features are exertional dyspnoea, cyanosis, and finger clubbing. In about 30% of cases, a bruit is audible over the site of the fistula. The malformations may bleed, leading to haemoptysis (as in this case) or intrapulmonary haemorrhage.

B In 30–60% of patients with pulmonary arteriovenous malformations, they occur as part of the syndrome of hereditary haemorrhagic telangiectasia, the 'Osler–Rendu–Weber syndrome'. There are visible telangiectatic lesions most easily seen on the face particularly around the mouth (2). Bleeding can occur from such lesions wherever they may be, in the form of epistaxis and gastrointestinal haemorrhage, for example.

C Arterial blood gases reveal an oxygen saturation that ranges from 50–90%, consequent to a potential right-to-left shunt. There is often associated polycythaemia, and anaemia due to haemorrhage can also occur. In over 90% of cases, the pulmonary arteriovenous malformation is visible on the chest radiograph as a rounded opacity in the lung field; the feeding and draining vessels may also be visible. Contrast echocardiography is useful in confirming a right-to-left shunt; if the contrast is injected in the pulmonary artery and detected in the left atrium, the intrapulmonary shunt is confirmed. Computer tomographic (CT) scanning may also reveal pulmonary arteriovenous malformations by using contrast enhancement or ultrafast (cine) CT. Pulmonary scintigraphy and magnetic resonance imaging may also prove useful diagnostic aids.

D The prognosis of pulmonary arteriovenous malformation is generally good, but it may cause considerable disability, especially consequent to haemorrhagic events. Rarely, paradoxical embolism into the systemic circulation or cerebral abscess formation can occur, with potentially fatal results.

E If there is significant clinical disability from an isolated malformation it can be resected. Alternatively, it is often possible to obstruct the malformation with detachable balloons or metal coils introduced via the systemic venous system. These latter techniques may prove difficult, however, if the malformation is complex and has multiple feeding vessels.

Reference

Dines DE, Sewart JB, Bernatza PE. Pulmonary arteriovenous fistulas. *Proc Mayo Clin* 1983; **58**:176-181.

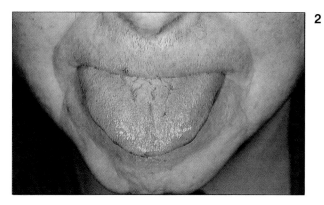

2 Visible telangiectatic lesions seen around the mouth and on the tongue in a patient with Osler–Rendu–Weber syndrome.

Case 15

An important cause of palpitations

History

A 19-year-old woman presented with palpitations and an episode of pre-syncope. She had previously experienced occasional mild palpitations. The electrocardiogram at admission is shown in (1). The patient was given intravenous lignocaine but her electrocardiogram remained unchanged. Synchronized DC cardioversion resulted in restoration of sinus rhythm (2). Clinical examination was entirely normal. An echocardiogram was reported as normal.

Questions

A What do the electrocardiograms (1 and 2) show?
B Comment on the management of such arrhythmias.
C What further investigations should be performed?
D What future treatment regimen would you recommend?

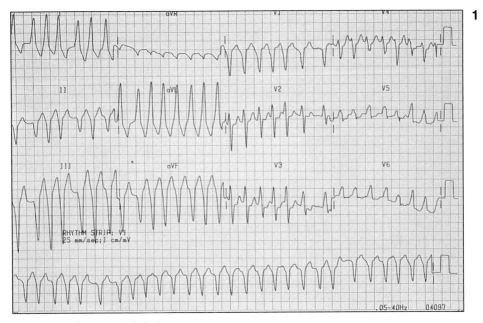

1 Electrocardiogram at admission.

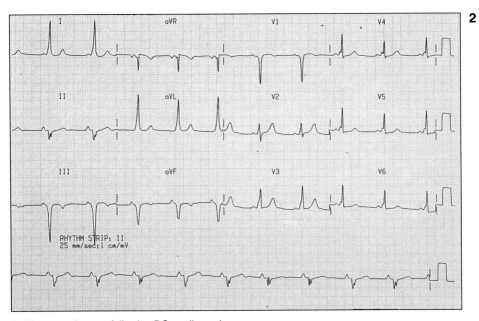

2 Electrocardiogram following DC cardioversion.

Case 15

Answers

A The electrocardiogram (1) shows a broad complex tachycardia. The QRS complex is predominantly negative in lead V_1 (left bundle branch block-like pattern), which often makes it difficult to distinguish between ventricular and supraventricular tachycardia. There is great irregularity in the RR interval, however, suggesting that the rhythm is likely to be supraventricular (the RR interval during ventricular tachycardia seldom varies by more than 40ms), possibly atrial fibrillation with bundle branch block or pre-excitation. (2) shows the 12-lead electrocardiogram in sinus rhythm. It demonstrates the 'Wolff–Parkinson–White' (WPW) pattern, with a short PR interval and wide QRS with an initial slurred component (delta wave). The classification of bypass tracts in this condition was originally type A (positive delta wave in V_1) and type B (negative delta wave in V_1, as in this case), associated with left- and right-side pre-excitation, respectively. Currently, atrioventricular bypass tracts are thought to occur in one of four general locations (**Table 1**), defined by studying the 12-lead electrocardiogram and by intracardiac mapping in the electrophysiology laboratory.

B The marked irregularity of the RR interval makes ventricular tachycardia extremely unlikely, and therefore lignocaine is not an appropriate anti-arrhythmic agent in this case. While synchronized DC cardioversion was successful, medical cardioversion should be considered when it is likely that atrial fibrillation is present. Although quinidine has been widely used for medical cardioversion of atrial fibrillation (success rate of 65–85%), it can increase the ventricular response in some cases. Flecainide lengthens intra-arterial, atrioventricular and intraventricular conduction (increasing the duration of PR interval and QRS complex), and is effective in terminating atrioventricular nodal re-entrant tachycardias due to an accessory pathway. It is also effective in pre-excited atrial fibrillation, terminating the arrhythmia in 50% of cases.

C Atrial fibrillation associated with the WPW syndrome may be life threatening if the accessory pathway has a short refractory period, allowing a very rapid ventricular rate. Ventricular fibrillation may result if the antegrade impulse reaches the ventricles during the 'vulnerable period'. Atrial fibrillation should therefore be induced during an electrophysiology study and the shortest pre-excited RR interval measured. If the RR intervals are shorter than 250ms, long-term antiarrhythmic therapy should be administered.

D The most common prophylactic treatment for potentially lethal bypass tracts is to administer drugs that increase the antegrade refractory period of the bypass tract (e.g. Class Ic drugs such as flecainide). If drug therapy is inadequate or if life-long drug therapy is undesirable, ablation of the tract should be strongly considered. In this case of a posteroseptal bypass tract, transcatheter radio-frequency ablation can be considered as an alternative to surgery.

Location of tract	Characteristics of pre-excited QRS
Left free wall	Right free wall
Posteroseptal	Anteroseptal
Q wave, lateral precordial leads	LBBB, superior axis
Q wave, inferior leads	LBBB, inferior axis

Table 1 Localization of bypass tracts by findings on the 12-lead electrocardiogram.

A cause of hypertension

History

A 19-year-old woman was found to be hypertensive (180/100mmHg) and to have a 'heart murmur' at a medical examination for employment purposes. She denied any symptoms and there was no relevant medical history. A chest radiograph (1) was performed and, as a result, the patient was referred to a cardiologist.

Questions

A   What does the chest radiograph (1) show?
B   What physical signs may be present in this patient?
C   What other cardiovascular problems are associated with this condition?
D   What further investigations are required?
E   What treatment should this patient be offered?

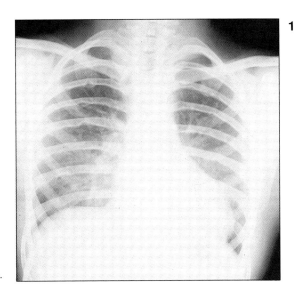

1

1 Chest radiograph appearance.

Case 16

Answers

A   The chest radiograph (1) reveals cardiac enlargement (cardiothoracic ratio = 12/22) with left ventricular prominence. The inferior surfaces of the 4th–9th ribs show indentations with sclerotic margins. The appearances are due to coarctation of the aorta with dilated intercostal arteries. Note that 'rib notching' does not occur in the first and second ribs as the first two intercostals do not arise from the aorta. The constriction is usually eccentric, distal to the left subclavian artery, opposite the ductus arteriosus (termed 'juxta ductal').

B   The patient will be hypertensive and this may involve the right ± the left arm (depending on whether the left subclavian is involved). The femoral pulses are likely to be weak, delayed or even absent. There may be noticeable carotid and subclavian pulsations, and collaterals may be palpable around the shoulders and scapulae. Murmurs occur from the coarctation and may be continuous or ejection systolic. They may also occur from the collateral vessels and be due to the association with a bicuspid aortic valve (approximately 50% of cases).

C   Associated cardiac lesions are common with the infantile type of coarctation (including patent ductus arteriosus, ventricular septal defect, transposition of the great arteries), but these are much less common in the adult type seen here (with the exception of a bicuspid aortic valve). Infective endocarditis can occur on the coarctation or bicuspid valve. Rupture or dissection of the proximal aorta (especially in pregnancy), angina pectoris (premature coronary disease) and left ventricular failure can all be present in this condition.

D   Cross-sectional echocardiography (from the suprasternal notch) can visualize the aortic arch and proximal descending aorta in children and adolescents, but in older patients the image is often of insufficient quality to allow confident diagnosis. From this position, however, the continuous wave Doppler transducer can be angled to direct its beam parallel to the descending aortic flow. The velocity waveform recorded may vary, though. In patients with mild obstruction and no collaterals, the high-velocity jet produced is restricted to systole. With increasing severity of coarctation, the high-velocity jet spills over into diastole. With a very severe coarctation, flow is continuous with an incomplete pressure equalization even in late diastole (2). This diastolic flow may represent flow across a severe coarctation or may originate from collateral flow. With a good-quality signal and trans-coarctation flow restricted to systole, accurate assessment of the pressure drop can be obtained. When flow is prolonged into diastole, however, the accuracy of the technique diminishes and gradient underestimation can occur.

Digital subtraction arch aortography provides visualization of the site of the coarctation and the length of affected aorta, but no haemodynamic information. The site of coarctation can also be effectively shown using magnetic resonance imaging (MRI). Haemodynamic evaluation may require invasive investigation by retrograde cardiac catheterization via the femoral artery or combined with a brachial arteriotomy if the coarctation cannot be crossed. The findings include left ventricular and ascending aortic hypertension with a lower pressure and pulse volume in the descending aorta. A coarctation gradient of 40mmHg is highly significant. Aortography allows the site of coarctation and the collateral circulation to be visualized.

E   There is no effective medical treatment for coarctation. Surgical resection and end-to-end anastomosis is often performed, although balloon dilatation is increasingly advocated, as in this case (3–5). Aneurysmal expansion following dilatation can occur, however. Relief of hypertension follows either procedure, although some patients require antihypertensive agents for a variable period of time and a few remain hypertensive even with medication. Recoarctation can also occur and this is often dealt with by balloon dilatation.

Reference

Morrow WR, Vick GW, Nihill MR, et al. Balloon dilatation of unoperated coarctation of the aorta: short and intermediate results. *J Am Coll Cardiol* 1988; **11**:133-138.

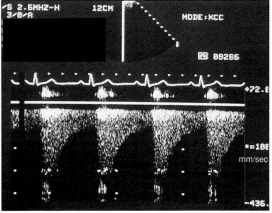

2 The descending aortic flow (suprasternal approach) profile in a patient with severe coarctation. The waveform indicates that high-velocity flow takes place in diastole as well as systole.

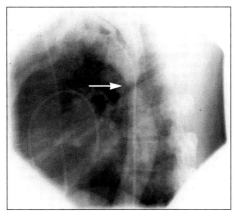

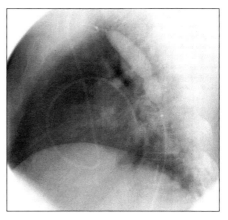

3 The aortogram before balloon angioplasty, showing a discrete constriction just distal to the left subclavian artery (arrow).

4 Balloon angioplasty at the coarctation site. Note the balloon 'waisting'.

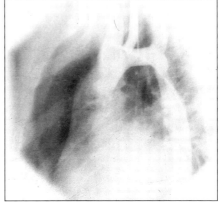

5 After angioplasty there is only mild narrowing at the coarctation site.

Case 17

Exercise-induced arrhythmia

History

A 40-year-old woman was referred by her general practitioner with a history of recurrent dizzy spells and palpitations related to exertion. She had recently been discharged from a local psychiatric hospital following treatment for depression. Clinical examination was normal. An electrocardiogram was taken (1) and the patient underwent an exercise stress test. This was abruptly stopped when the patient experienced palpitations and pre-syncope. The electrocardiogram at this stage is shown in (2).

Questions

A What do the electrocardiograms (1 and 2) show?
B What is the likely cause of this patient's symptoms?
C How would you manage this patient?

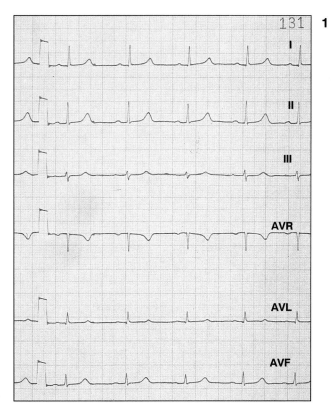

1 Resting electrocardiogram.

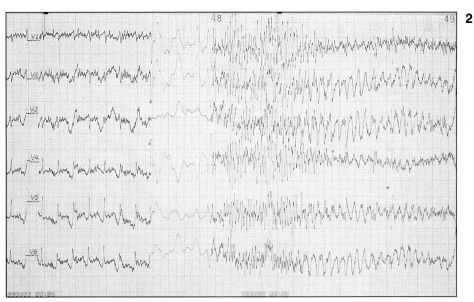

2 Exercise electrocardiogram.

Case 17

Answers

A The exercise electrocardiogram (2) shows sinus rhythm degenerating into a very rapid rate, with abnormally wide, abnormally shaped QRS complexes. Furthermore, there is rhythmic shifting of the cardiac axis so that the QRS complexes appear tall for a few beats and then shorter. This is an unusual, polymorphic form of ventricular tachycardia sometimes called '*torsades de pointes*', literally 'twisting of the points'. The arrhythmia is frequently self-limiting and repeats for 5–10 seconds at a time. It usually arises on the background of a prolonged QT interval. The QT interval normally shortens with increasing heart rate and can be corrected for heart rate (QT_c) by dividing the measured interval by the square root of the cycle length. The normal QT_c is less than 420ms and in this case is 450ms. The combination of *torsades de pointes* and a long QT interval is known as 'long QT syndrome' (**Table 1**).

B The patient had recently been admitted with a severe depressive illness associated with an anxiety state and had been given large doses of chlorpromazine. She was also taking imipramine. It is likely that the combination of the phenothiazine with a tricyclic antidepressant resulted in long QT syndrome in this case. The patient's electrolytes should be carefully checked, looking for depletion of potassium, calcium or magnesium (all of which are also potential causes of long QT syndrome).

C The withdrawal of chlorpromazine and/or imipramine is mandatory and in this case was covered by the short-term use of diazepam and subsequent introduction of a non-cyclical antidepressant. The ventricular arrhythmia settled over 2 weeks and the QT_c interval shortened to 318ms. Subsequent Holter monitoring and a repeat exercise stress test showed no further arrhythmia.

Congenital

    Jervell and Lange–Nielson syndrome

    (associated with congenital deafness)

    Romano–Ward syndrome

Acquired

    Drugs:

        Class I and III antiarrhythmics

        Tricyclic antidepressants

        Phenothiazines

    Metabolic abnormalities:

        Hypokalaemia

        Hypomagnesaemia

        Hypocalcaemia

    Cardiac abnormalities:

        Myocardial infarction

        Mitral valve prolapse

        Significant bradycardia

Table 1 Causes of long QT syndrome.

Endocarditis and change in bowel habit

History

A 64-year-old male presented with malaise and weight loss. There was a long history of vague abdominal pain and intermittant change in bowel habit. On examination the patient was pyrexial (38.2°C) with tachycardia and a loud pansystolic murmur was heard at the apex.

Investigations: Hb 9.1 g/dL, white cell count 12×10^6, ESR 94mm/hr. Blood culture grew *Streptococcus bovis* in all 6 bottles.

Question

A Given that this patient presented with *Streptococcus bovis* endocarditis of the mitral valve, what investigations are necessary over and above the normal management of bacterial endocarditis?

Answer

A This organism is usually associated with gastrointestinal (GI) tract pathology, and bacterial endocarditis can be the first presenting manifestation. Barium studies of the lower GI tract should therefore be performed at a suitable interval, with appropriate antibiotic cover (1).

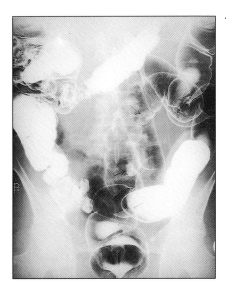

1

1 Barium enema examination in this patient, demonstrating an extensive colonic polyp.

Case 19

Arrhythmia following myocardial infarction

History

A 50-year-old man presented with palpitations associated with dizziness and shortness of breath. He had suffered an acute myocardial infarction 9 months previously, which was complicated by an episode of severe acute left ventricular failure. He was taking frusemide 80mg once daily and captopril 12.5mg tds at the time of representation. The pulse was approximately 150 beats per minute and blood pressure was 120/90mmHg. There was no evidence of heart failure. An electrocardiogram (1) and chest radiograph (2) were taken. The patient was given lignocaine 100mg intravenously without effect on the arrhythmia. Synchronized DC cardioversion was then performed and the patient reverted to sinus rhythm (3). Cardiac enzymes remained normal.

Questions

A   What do the electrocardiograms (1 and 3) show?
B   What does the chest radiograph (2) show?
C   What further investigations should be performed in this case?
D   What treatment schedule should this patient be offered?

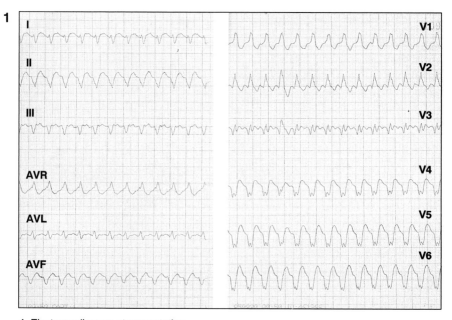

1 Electrocardiogram at presentation.

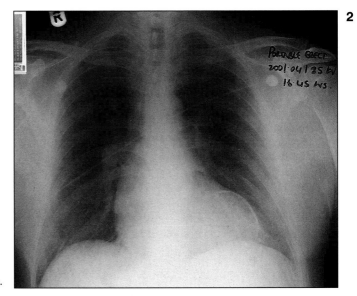

2 Chest radiograph.

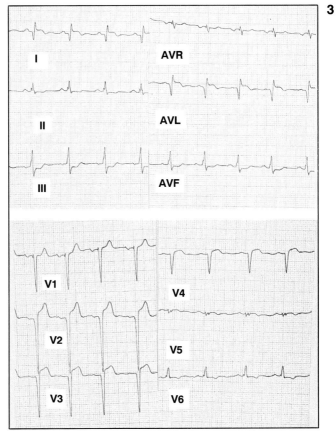

3 Electrocardiogram in sinus rhythm.

Case 19

Answers

A The electrocardiogram (1) shows a broad complex tachycardia. Several arrhythmias may produce such an appearance – ventricular tachycardia, supraventricular tachycardia with rate-related aberrant conduction, and any supraventricular tachycardia in a patient with pre-existing bundle branch block or pre-excitation. In this case the rhythm is regular, the QRS duration is greater than140ms, there is evidence of atrioventricular dissociation, left axis deviation and a right bundle branch block pattern in V_1 with an Rsr' configuration. These electrocardiographic features are highly suggestive of ventricular tachycardia. Patients with ischaemic heart disease are more likely to develop such arrhythmias. In some patients an atrial electrocardiogram, recorded simultaneously with a surface ECG, is necessary to demonstrate independent atrial activity (4). This can be obtained by passing a transvenous electrode to the right atrium or by using an oesophageal electrode positioned behind the left atrium. The electrocardiogram in sinus rhythm (3) shows an extensive antero-lateral myocardial infarction with persistence of the pattern of acute infarction long after recovery, suggesting the existence of an extensive fibrous scar in the ventricular wall associated with aneurysm formation.

B The chest radiograph (2) is a portable film. Nevertheless, there is cardiomegaly with left ventricular prominence. There is extensive calcification in a probable ventricular aneurysm, some of which is probably in mural clot.

C Cross-sectional echocardiography (5) allows visualization of ventricular aneurysms in most cases. It also provides information on mural thrombi and the state of the remaining myocardium, an important appraisal if surgery is being considered. However, the best non-invasive method for visualizing a ventricular aneurysm is probably nuclear electro-cardiographic gated blood pool imaging (usually using Technetium-99m). Cardiac catheterization may be necessary to demonstrate the coronary arteries and left ventricular angiography can be performed at the same time (although the latter may produce embolization of mural thrombus). The inducibility or non-inducibility of ventricular tachycardia is also of prime importance in such a case. Exercise testing should be used in the initial assessment to document the likelihood of exercise inducing the tachycardia and the relationship between ischaemia and the tachycardia. Programmed electrical stimulation should ideally be performed and electrical 'mapping' of the myocardium may define a trigger zone which could be resected surgically.

D The first line of treatment for ventricular tachyarrhythmia is antiarrhythmic drug therapy. Ideally, an electrophysiology study is used to identify effective therapy. If a ventricular arrhythmia that was inducible during baseline (drug-free) testing is no longer inducible after administering a drug, then that drug has probably had a favourable effect (on the re-entrant circuit). Chronic treatment with that drug can be expected to be effective in preventing further clinical arrhythmia. It is not practical, however, to perform such investigations in every patient. The left ventricular aneurysm was thought to be too extensive for surgical resection in this case, and coronary angiography showed single vessel disease (proximal occlusion of the left anterior descending artery). The patient was treated with amiodarone and had no further arrhythmia whilst maintained on this therapy (normal 24-hour Holter monitoring).

References

Dancy M, Ward D. Diagnosis of ventricular tachycardia: a clinical algorithm. *Br Med J* 1985; 291:1036-1038.

Visser CA, Kon G, Meltzer RS, *et al*. Incidence, timing and prognostic value of left ventricular aneurysm formation after infarction. *Am J Cardiol* 1986; 57:729-732.

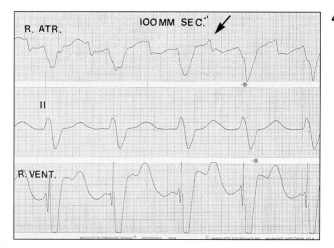

4 Lead II recorded at 100mm/sec with right atrial (R. ATR.) and right ventricular (R. VENT.) electrograms. Atrial activity (arrow) is independent of ventricular activity, indicating ventricular tachycardia.

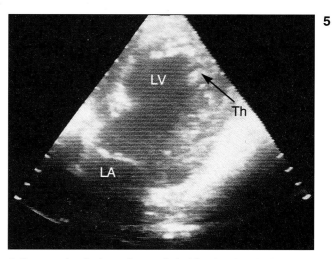

5 Cross-sectional echocardiogram (apical fourchamber view) showing a large left ventricular aneurysm, containing a thrombus. The 'hinge point' is clearly visible. LA, left atrium; LV, left ventricle; Th, thrombus.

An unusual cause of angina and shortness of breath

History

A 50-year-old woman was referred by her general practitioner, with breathlessness and attacks of paroxysmal nocturnal dyspnoea. She also complained of intermittent chest pain on exertion, with relief by rest. Her GP had prescribed sublingual glyceryl trinitrate, which led to some relief of her symptoms. On examination the pulse was of good volume, in sinus rhythm. Blood pressure was 140/75mmHg. The apex beat was heaving and displaced laterally. Auscultation revealed a fourth heart sound and a grade 3/6 pan-systolic murmur at the apex which radiated to the axilla. The electrocardiogram showed left ventricular hypertrophy with T-wave inversion in the antero-lateral leads. A chest radiograph revealed cardiomegaly and changes of pulmonary plethora in the lung fields. Cross-sectional and M-mode echocardiography was performed (1, 2 and 3) and the patient subsequently underwent cardiac catheterization.

Questions

A   What abnormalities are seen in the echocardiograms (1, 2 and 3)?
B   What further investigations should be performed?
C   (4) shows the left heart catheter pressures. What abnormalities are seen and what do they reflect?
D   (5) shows the left ventricular angiogram from the catheter study. What does it indicate?
E   What treatment regimen should be recommended for this condition?

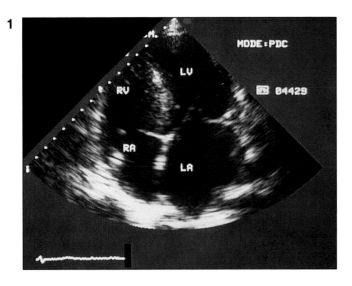

1 Cross-sectional echo-cardiogram from the apical four-chamber view. RV, right ventricle; LV, left ventricle; RA, right atrium; LA, left atrium.

2

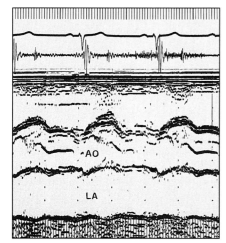

3

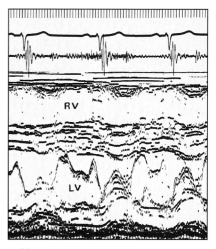

2 M-mode echocardiogram (parasternal long-axis view) with phonocardiogram. AO, aorta; LA, left atrium.

3 M-mode echocardiogram (together with phonocardiogram) from the parasternal long-axis view. RV, right ventricle; LV, left ventricle.

4

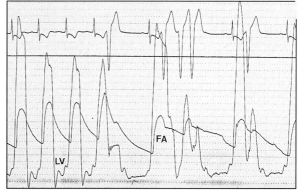

4 Left ventricular (LV) and femoral artery (FA) pressure tracings (0–200mmHg range).

5

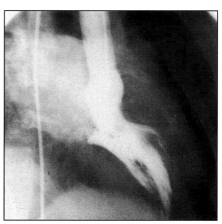

5 End-systolic frame from a left ventricular angiogram in the 30° right anterior oblique projection.

Case 20

Answers

A   The most striking abnormality is gross asymmetric septal hypertrophy (1 and 3), which is a sensitive (but not specific) echocardiographic feature in hypertrophic cardiomyopathy. There is also systolic anterior movement of the anterior mitral leaflet (3) which correlates well with the presence of outflow tract obstruction of the left ventricle. This is an important feature associated with changes in left ventricular shape when the left ventricular cavity becomes small or partly obliterated. This change in shape probably also contributes to mitral regurgitation, a frequent occurrence in hypertrophic cardiomyopathy. Partial mid-systolic closure of the aortic valve (2) is another characteristic feature of hypertrophic obstructive cardiomyopathy and again correlates with left ventricular outflow tract obstruction.

B   Doppler ultrasound can be used to demonstrate the degree of outflow obstruction and the presence of mitral regurgitation. Doppler-calculated gradients correlate well with those measured invasively. It is therefore not usually necessary nowadays to perform cardiac catheterization to diagnose hypertrophic cardiomyopathy, unless symptoms are refractory or there is doubt concerning the severity of mitral regurgitation. However, cardiac catheterization for the purpose of performing coronary arteriography is often required in patients over 40 years of age who have significant angina.

C   In this case there is a pressure gradient at rest between the left ventricle and femoral artery which has increased following an extrasystolic beat. On catheter withdrawal from the left ventricle, the pressure gradient was demonstrated between the body and outflow tract of the left ventricle (not shown). In a small proportion of patients, a right ventricular infundibular gradient may also be demonstrated. The coronary arteries were normal in this patient.

D   Left ventricular angiography (5) reveals an abnormally formed ventricle ('banana shaped') which ejects at least 75% of its contents in association with severe mitral regurgitation. The papillary muscles are very prominent and obliterate the left ventricular cavity in late systole.

E   In many patients with hypertrophic cardiomyopathy pharmacological treatment alone will improve symptoms. Beta-adrenoceptor blockers (especially propranolol) and calcium antagonists (particularly verapamil) provide increased time for left ventricular filling by blunting the heart rate response (especially during exercise), and reduce the left ventricular gradient through a negative inotropic effect. In this case, because of the presence of severe mitral regurgitation associated with a large left ventricular outflow tract gradient, the patient underwent cardiac surgery. A segment of the upper anterior septum was removed (myotomy/myectomy) and the mitral valve replaced. This resulted in symptomatic and haemodynamic benefit.

Arrhythmia is a common complication of hypertrophic cardiomyopathy and amiodarone is effective in suppressing supraventricular (atrial fibrillation or supraventricular tachycardia) or ventricular arrhythmia. This drug is also associated with improved survival when compared to matched control subjects consequent to suppression of ventricular arrhythmia. In this case no arrhythmias were demonstrated on ambulatory Holter monitoring.

Reference

McKenna WJ. Hypertrophic cardiomyopathy. In: *Diseases of the heart*. Julian DG, Camm AJ, Fox KM, Hall RJC, Poole-Wilson PA (eds). London: Baillière Tindall, 1989.

Cardiovascular complications from a rheumatology clinic

History

A 50-year-old man with chronic low back pain and 'arthritis' of the hips and knees was referred to a cardiologist because a heart murmur was noted. The patient denied any cardiovascular symptoms. On examination, the patient was apyrexial with no peripheral signs of infective endocarditis. Blood pressure was 160/90mmHg. There was no evidence of cardiomegaly or heart failure, but a diastolic murmur was heard. A cross-sectional/M-mode echocardiogram was taken (1 and 2) and the patient's X-rays (3) were reviewed.

Questions

A   What does the echocardiogram (1 and 2) show?
B   What is the cause of the patient's back pain?
C   By what likely mechanism has the heart murmur developed?
D   What other cardiovascular complications can occur in this rheumatological condition?

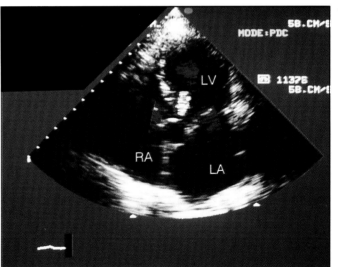

1 Cross-sectional echocardiogram in the apical four-chamber view with colour-flow imaging. LV, left ventricle; LA, left atrium; RA, right atrium.

Case 21

2

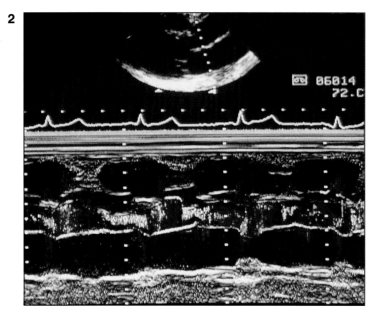

2 M-mode echo-cardiogram (para-sternal long axis view) with colour-flow imaging.

3

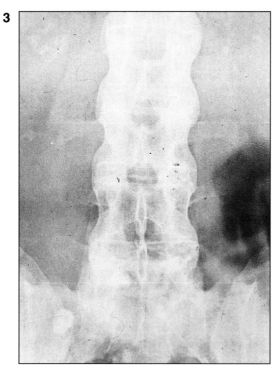

3 Lumbar spine X-ray of patient.

Answers

A (1) shows a cross-sectional echocardiogram in the apical four-chamber view with colour-flow imaging. The diastolic frame exhibits turbulence (orange and blue signal) in the left ventricular outflow tract produced by a regurgitant jet which originates from the aortic valve. (2) is a colour-flow M-mode echocardiogram (parasternal long axis view) showing, again, a diastolic turbulant regurgitant jet originating from the aortic valve. The appearances are those of aortic regurgitation.

B The lumbar spine X-ray (3) shows classic features of long-standing ankylosing spondylitis, with squaring of the vertebral bodies, calcification of the interspinous ligaments, plus sclerosis and ankylosis of the apophyseal joints. This produces the characteristic radiological appearance of the 'bamboo spine'.

C In patients with long-standing ankylosing spondylitis inflammation and scarring of the aortic valve and wall of the aorta immediately above the valve occur. The result is aortitis, dilatation of the valve ring and scarring of the aortic valve cusps, leading to aortic regurgitation, which may be severe. The prevalence of clinically recognized aortic regurgitation is low, however, possibly affecting only 1–2% of patients with ankylosing spondylitis. The inflammatory process also occasionally spreads to the base of the anterior cusp of the mitral valve, producing mitral regurgitation.

D The other classic cardiac manifestation of ankylosing spondylitis is heart block produced by extension of the inflammatory process into the muscular interventricular septum, thereby damaging the His bundle and its branches. This may give rise to bundle branch block as well as atrioventricular block of all degrees. Furthermore, aortic regurgitation and heart block often coexist. Permanent pacing may be required in selected cases.

Reference

Ansell BM, Bywaters EG, Doniach I. The aortic lesion of ankylosing spondylitis. *Br Heart J* 1958; **20**:507-515.

Case 22

A forgotten cardiovascular disease

History

An 18-year-old student presented with a 3-week history of sweating, anorexia and listlessness, together with a 1-week history of pain and stiffness in his knees and ankles. There was no history of sore throat. Examination revealed a temperature of 38°C and the patient was pale. Inspection of the trunk revealed a rash which the patient had not noticed (1). The knees and ankles were painful on movement but there was no swelling or excessive warmth on palpation. Cardiovascular examination was unremarkable. An electrocardiogram was taken (2).

Questions

A   What is the most likely diagnosis in this case?
B   What further investigations are required?
C   What treatment would you advise?

1

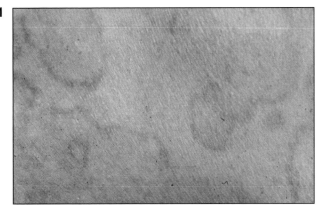

1 Truncal appearance of rash.

2

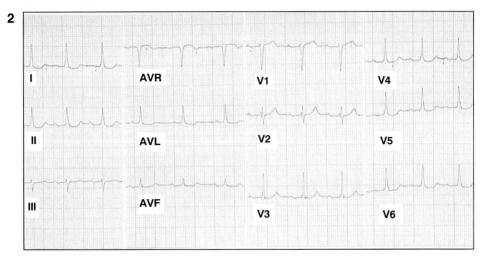

2 Electrocardiogram at presentation.

Answers

A The rash (1) consists of pink circumscribed circles with pale centres. The lesions are painless and do not itch. This is a classic sign of erythema marginatum, which is characteristic of rheumatic fever (although it has been reported in staphylococcal sepsis and in drug reactions). It usually affects the trunk and proximal extremities and may appear and disappear within hours. The electrocardiogram shows first degree atrioventricular block (PR interval 240ms). There is a history of fever and arthralgia. A diagnosis of rheumatic fever is, therefore, likely, provided evidence of streptococcal infection can be obtained (**Table 1**).

Major criteria	Minor criteria	Evidence of streptococcal infection
Polyarthritis	Arthralgia	Positive throat culture
Carditis	Fever	Raised antistreptolysin O
Chorea	Previous rheumatic fever	and other antibody titres
Erythema marginatum	Prolonged PR interval	Recent scarlet fever
Subcutaneous nodules	Elevated acute phase	
	reactants (white cell count,	
	ESR, C-reactive protein)	

Table 1 Duckett Jones criteria for the diagnosis of rheumatic fever. For diagnosis, two major criteria or one major and two minor criteria, plus evidence of streptococcal infection, are required.

B A history of sore throat occurs in 60% of sufferers; this patient had no such history and a throat swab was negative. Blood cultures should be performed but the diagnosis of rheumatic fever is usually confirmed by a raised antistreptolysin O antibody titre. Although non-specific, evidence of an elevated white cell count, ESR and C-reactive protein should be sought, together with any sign of normochromic normocytic anaemia. Daily auscultation of the precordium should be performed. An apical soft pan-systolic murmur was heard a few days after hospital admission in this patient.

C During the acute phase of illness bed rest is recommended. Salicylates and corticosteroids are useful for relief of symptoms but there is little evidence that they shorten the course of the acute illness or prevent progression to chronic valvular disease. Patients do require penicillin, however, to prevent recurrence and this should be continued for at least 5 years or until the patient reaches his or her early 20s (whichever is the longest).

Reference

Jones criteria (revised) for guidance in the diagnosis of rheumatic fever. *Circulation* 1965; 32:664-668.

Case 23

An unusual cause of palpitations

History

A 68-year-old man presented with a sudden onset of palpitations and dizziness. Electrocardiography was performed (1) and the rhythm required DC cardioversion. Once sinus rhythm had been restored, physical examination showed a raised jugular venous pressure with a prominent 'a' wave and a positive Kussmaul's sign. The pulse was 80 beats per minute and blood pressure 160/90mmHg. Auscultation of the precordium revealed a third heart sound followed by a low-pitched mid-diastolic murmur and a harsh pan-systolic murmur loudest at the left sternal edge. All laboratory test results were normal except those for total bilirubin, 36nmol/l and, lactate dehydrogenase, 479IU/l. The electrocardiogram following cardioversion revealed sinus rhythm with first degree atrioventricular block. The chest radiograph showed mild cardiomegaly.

Questions

A   What is the most likely underlying diagnosis?
B   What single investigation would you perform to confirm this?
C   What does the initial electrocardiogram (1) show, and what electrocardiographic abnormalities may occur?
D   What is the likely cause of the third heart sound in this case?
E   What is the likely cause of the biochemical abnormalities?

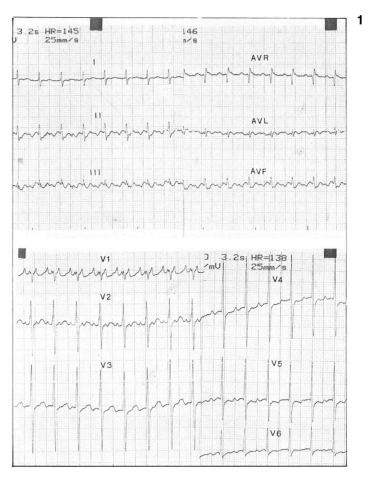

1 Electrocardiogram at initial presentation.

Case 23

Answers

A   A large 'a' wave with raised jugular venous pressure may be seen in any condition in which there is increased resistance to right atrial emptying and hence augmented atrial systole. This may occur in tricuspid stenosis or obstruction at tricuspid valve level by right atrial 'tumour'. Any cause of right ventricular hypertrophy, e.g. pulmonary hypertension, will also result in an increased 'a' wave in the venous pulse. It may additionally be seen in conditions associated with left ventricular hypertrophy. The associated positive Kussmaul's sign (a rise in venous pressure during inspiration) suggests mechanical impairment of venous return and makes intermittent obstruction due to right atrial tumour likely. This would explain the heart murmurs in this case.

B   The most appropriate investigation is echocardiography. (2) and (3) show M-mode and cross-sectional images, respectively, from this patient. (2) demonstrates a mass of echoes behind the tricuspid valve; these fill the right ventricular chamber during diastole and produce paradoxical posterior bulging of the interventricular septum. The abnormal echoes disappear during ventricular systole. Cross-sectional echocardiography (3) demonstrates a large mobile tumour mass in the right atrium which originates from the interatrial septum and prolapses into the right ventricle in diastole, distorting the interventricular septum. The right atrium and ventricle are dilated but the left atrium and ventricle are normal.

At operation a large gelatinous globular mass originating from the fossa ovalis was successfully removed. Histology confirmed the tumour to be a benign atrial myxoma.

C   Both paroxysmal and sustained supraventricular arrhythmia, particularly atrial flutter (in this case with 2:1 atrioventricular block (1)) or fibrillation, have been reported with right atrial myxoma. Right atrial and right ventricular hypertrophy also occur as can right bundle branch block and right axis deviation. First degree atrioventricular block was present in this case but resolved post-operatively, suggesting possible mechanical effects on the underlying conduction tissue by vigorous movements of the prolapsing tumour mass.

D   The third sound is likely to be an audible 'tumour plop' produced as the myxoma is hurled vigorously against intracardiac structures in various phases of the cardiac cycle. In this case the impact force was sufficient to distort the normal shape of the interventricular septum, a substantial structure.

E   The elevated lactate dehydrogenase and total bilirubin may be due to red cell destruction resulting from contact with the uneven surfaces of the tumour. Red cell morphology and the presence of damaged red cells were not evaluated in this case, however.

References

Massumi R. Bedside diagnosis of right heart myxomas through detection of palpable tumour shocks and audible plops. *Am Heart J* 1983; **105**:303-310.

Panidis IO, Kotler MN, Mintz GS, *et al.* Clinical and echocardiographic features of right atrial masses. *Am Heart J* 1984; **107**:745-748.

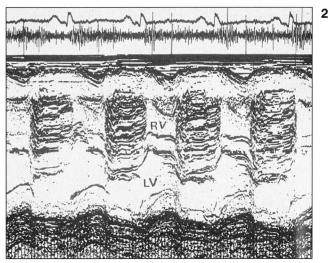

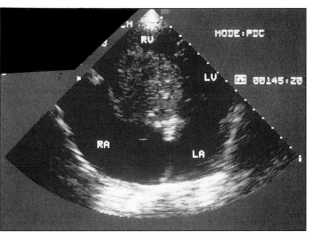

2 & 3 M-mode echocardio-gram (**2**) and cross-sectional echocardiogram (apical four-chamber view) (**3**). RV, right ventricle; RA, right atrium; LV, left ventricle; LA, left atrium.

Cardiology referral from a neurology clinic

History

A 40-year-old man was referred by a consultant neurologist to the cardiology clinic with a recent history of recurrent episodes of sudden loss of consciousness. The patient had experienced increasing difficulty in everyday activities over a number of years due to fatigue and shortness of breath. Cardiovascular examination was unremarkable. The patient's electrocardiogram is illustrated in (1) and his facial appearance in (2).

Questions

A   What does the electrocardiogram (1) show?
B   What underlying disorder does this patient's facial appearance suggest?
C   What cardiovascular complications can occur in this condition?
D   What further investigations and treatment should be undertaken?

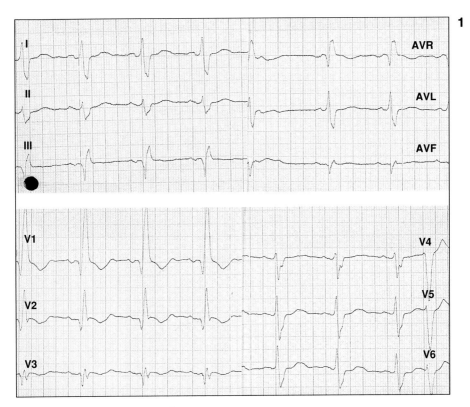

1 Electrocardiogram at presentation.

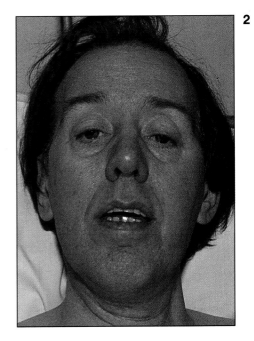

2 Facial appearance.

Case 24

Answers

A The electrocardiogram (1) shows sinus rhythm with a mean frontal plane axis of -15°. Normal initial 'r' waves are seen in the inferior leads, and the abnormal degree of left axis deviation therefore indicates the presence of left anterior hemiblock. The total QRS duration is prolonged beyond normal limits, i.e. RBBB pattern. This combination is thus a bifasicular block.

B The facial appearance is long and haggard, with facial myopathy, ptosis and frontal baldness. Such features are characteristic of dystrophia myotonia. This is a progressive multisystem disorder, inherited by an autosomal dominant gene, whose manifestations usually present in the third or fourth decade of life. Other features include distal muscular atrophy, cataracts, gonadal atrophy, impaired pulmonary ventilation and mental defect or dementia.

C Cardiac abnormalities frequently involve the conducting system in this disorder. These are more often recognized on the electrocardiogram than clinically and include sinus bradycardia, a tachy-brady syndrome, plus all types of atrioventricular and bundle branch block. In addition, the ECG may show repolarization abnormalities or a pseudo-infarction pattern. The heart may be enlarged and heart failure may occur. Respiratory involvement may produce hypoxaemia and pulmonary hypertension is possible.

D In this case, a 24-hour Holter recording was performed which showed episodes of 2:1 (Mobitz II) atrioventricular block. Therefore, a dual chamber permanent pacing system was implanted, which resolved the patient's episodes of loss of consciousness.

Reference

Davies MJ, Ward DE. The pathology of arrhythmias, conduction disturbances and sudden death. In: *Diseases of the heart.* Julian DG, Camm AJ, Fox KM, Hall RJC, Poole-Wilson PA (eds). London: Baillière Tindall, 1989.

An old electrocardiographic chestnut

History

A 70-year-old man presented to the casualty department with severe retrosternal chest pain which had lasted 2 hours. Clinical examination was normal and an electrocardiogram (1) was taken.

Questions

A   What does the electrocardiogram (1) show?
B   What further actions should be performed immediately ?

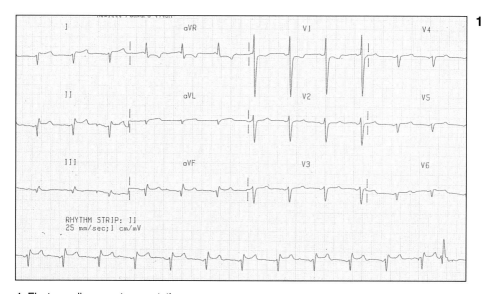

1 Electrocardiogram at presentation.

Case 25

Answers

A (1) shows abnormal Q waves and ST segment elevation in the infero-lateral leads consistent with a diagnosis of myocardial infarction. In addition, however, it should be noted that lead I is upside down, leads AVR and AVL are interchanged (arm leads transposed), leads II and III are interchanged (leg leads transposed), lead AVF is unaffected and there is progressive diminution in the size of the QRS complexes from V_1 to V_6. These changes are characteristic of dextrocardia inadvertently recorded with conventionally placed limb and chest leads. The trace may be mistaken for myocardial ischaemia with lateral infarction if the error is not realized. The real clue is the inverted 'P' wave in the antero-lateral leads, indicating that the sino-atrial node is not on the right-hand side of the heart. Inadvertent transposition of the arm leads in a normal subject mimics this tracing in many respects, but is readily differentiated by the normal contour of the chest leads.

B Interpretation of the electrocardiogram in cases of true dextrocardia has the usual meaning only if – as in this case – right and left arm connections are reversed and the precordial leads are reversed on the right side of the chest instead of the left (2). The diagnosis of inferior infarction is, of course, unaltered.

Reference

Rowlands DJ. *Understanding the electrocardiogram.* Section 2: Morphological abnormalities. London: ICI plc, 1982.

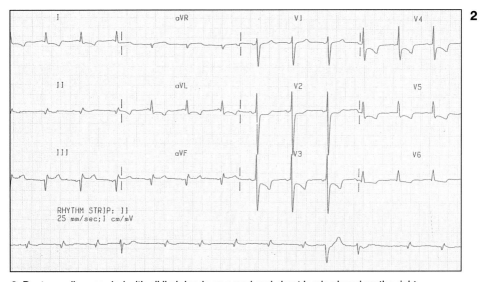

2 Dextrocardia recorded with all limb leads reversed and chest leads placed on the right.

Case 26

A case of persistent shortness of breath

History

A 56-year-old woman presented to her local hospital with a 6-hour history of progressive shortness of breath and cough. The patient had not experienced any chest pain. She had recently been diagnosed as mildly hypertensive by her general practitioner who had prescribed a thiazide diuretic. The medical registrar diagnosed acute left ventricular failure and initiated treatment with intravenous frusemide and diamorphine. Auscultation revealed a gallop rhythm and a soft pan-systolic murmur at the apex. The electrocardiogram showed sinus tachycardia and inverted T waves in leads V_5 and V_6. The patient's symptoms improved but 48 hours later she still had an increased respiratory rate, a sinus tachycardia and similar auscultatory findings. A repeat chest radiograph was taken (1). The cardiac enzymes were normal and the electrocardiogram was unchanged. Echocardiography (2) and a Swan Ganz catheter study (3) were performed.

Questions

A   Comment on the appearance of the repeat chest radiograph (1).
B   What diagnosis is suggested from the echocardiogram (2) and Swan Ganz catheter study (3)?
C   What further investigations (if any) should be performed in this case?
D   What treatment does this patient require?

1

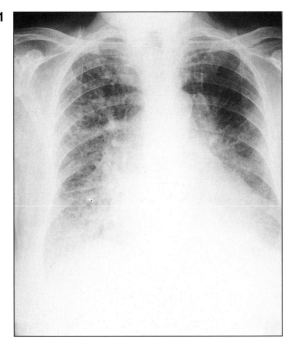

1 Chest radiograph 48 hours after presentation.

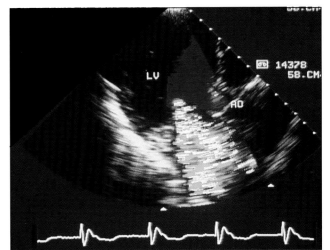

2 Apical two-chamber echo-cardiogram with colour-flow imaging taken in systole. LV, left ventricle; Ao, aorta.

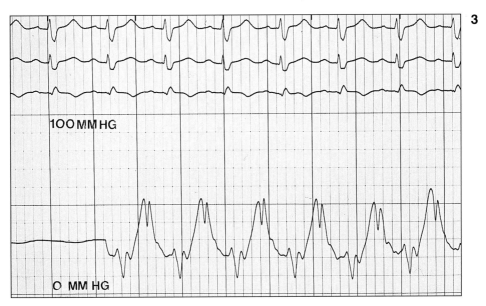

3 Pulmonary artery pressure tracing (0–100mmHg).

Case 26

Answers

A The appearance is consistent with alveolar pulmonary oedema. There is peripheral haze, thickening of the horizontal fissure and Kerley B lines are present. Consolidation is present in the lower zone.

B (2) shows a cross-sectional echocardiogram with colour-flow imaging in the apical two-chamber view. The left atrium contains multiple blue and yellow signals in systole, indicating a turbulent jet of mitral regurgitation. M-mode and cross-sectional echocardiography are poor methods of assessing the severity of mitral regurgitation, although they may reveal the underlying cause (**Table 1**). Continuous wave Doppler tracings may be useful in demonstrating the presence of mitral regurgitation, but quantification can also be difficult using this method. The width and depth of the signals by colour imaging indicate severe regurgitation in this case, although it should be remembered that this technique also has limited abilities as a quantitative tool. Right heart catheter (Swan Ganz) pressure measurements can be useful in indirectly assessing the severity of mitral regurgitation. There is usually a moderate degree of pulmonary hypertension (but the pulmonary artery pressure does not reach the levels often seen in severe mitral stenosis). (3) shows a pulmonary pressure of 50/20mmHg with superimposed backward transmission of the left atrial 'v' wave to the pulmonary artery ('giant 'v' wave'), suggesting severe mitral regurgitation.

C A left ventriculogram is extremely important in the assessment of mitral regurgitation. It demonstrates the reflux of dye from the left ventricle to the left atrium (4). The degree of mitral regurgitation can be assessed in two ways. Most commonly, a simple visual scale (usually out of 4) is used to determine whether the regurgitation is trivial, mild, moderate or severe. A more accurate and reproducible assessment can be obtained by calculating the regurgitant fraction, which is the amount of blood that regurgitates into the left atrium with each systole, expressed as a percentage of the total output of the left ventricle, i.e. the amount that regurgitates plus the amount that is ejected into the aorta with each systole. In this case the left ventricle contracts vigorously, and there is already complete opacification of the left atrium on the first systolic frame after the injection of contrast, indicating severe mitral regurgitation. Myocardial infarction should be excluded in this case, and coronary angiography is also required to delineate any related or incidental coronary artery disease in a patient of this age. In this case the coronary anatomy was normal.

D The presence of acute severe regurgitation requires urgent surgical correction. Prior to this being performed such patients can be beneficially supported with the use of vasodilators. Both arterial dilators, e.g. hydrallazine, and mixed arterial/venous dilators, e.g. glyceryl trinitrate or angiotensin converting enzyme (ACE) inhibitors, may prove useful for two reasons. First, reducing peripheral vascular resistance decreases left ventricular afterload and, therefore, some of the left ventricular output destined for the left atrium is redirected into the peripheral circulation. Secondly, the reduction in peripheral resistance reduces left ventricular size and, in combination with a reduction in pre-load, alters the degree of regurgitation by reducing the effective regurgitant orifice. The causes of acute mitral valve regurgitation are listed in **Table 1**. Cardiac surgery in this case revealed chordal rupture (spontaneous) affecting one-third of the anterior mitral leaflet. This was treated by excision and transfer of a segment of the posterior leaflet with its chordae to fill the defect. This procedure has a potential advantage in producing better haemodynamic function than replacing the mitral valve. This repair produced valve competence and the patient made an uneventful recovery.

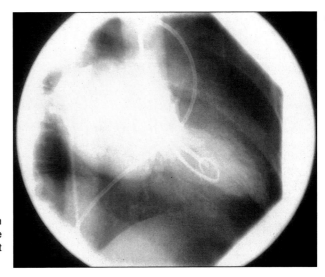

4 Left ventricular angiogram, on the first systolic frame after the injection of contrast (30° right anterior oblique projection).

Chordal rupture	Papillary muscle dysfunction	Cusp malfunction
Spontaneous or traumatic	Ischaemic	Mitral valve prolapse
Mitral valve prolapse	Following acute myocardial infarction	Perforation, e.g. by infective endocarditis
Infective endocarditis		

Table 1 Causes of acute mitral valve regurgitation.

Electrocardiographic diagnosis in cases of collapse

Questions

What diagnosis is suggested by the electrocardiogram in each of the following cases:

A   An 80-year-old woman was found collapsed at home (1).

B   A 70-year-old man collapsed while lifting up a bag of garden rubbish. He had recently had a permanent pacemaker fitted for complete heart block (2).

C   A 60-year-old man with dilated cardiomyopathy had a cardiac arrest. His drug treatment was frusemide, amiloride and captopril (3).

D   A 35-year-old woman who was thirty weeks pregnant presented with collapse (4).

E   A 50-year-old man presented with collapse and hypotension three days following coronary artery bypass surgery (5).

F   An 18-year-old girl, previously very well, presented with sudden collapse and was unconscious on arrival in casualty. There was no history of chest pain (6).

1

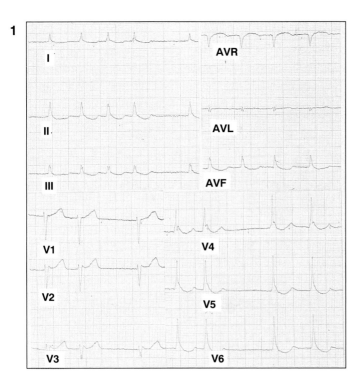

2

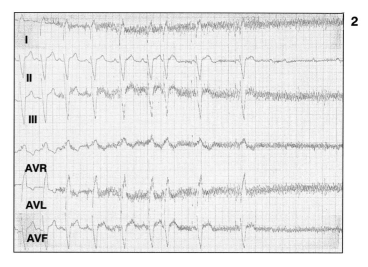

3

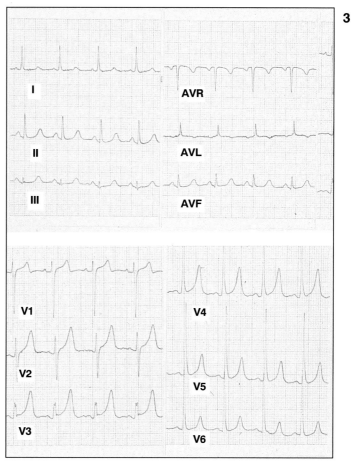

Case 27

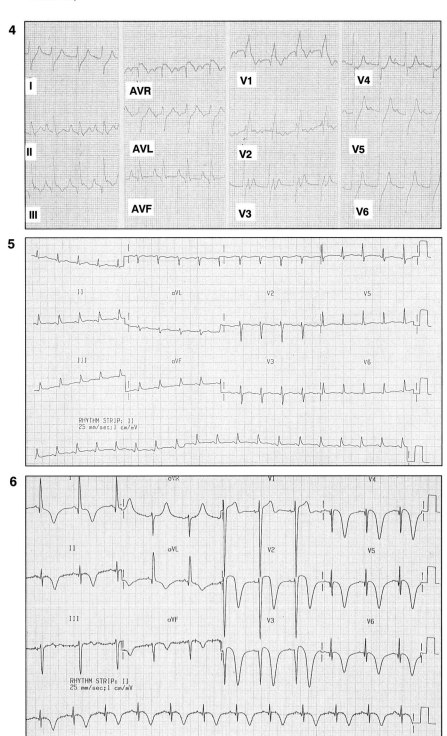

Answers

A *Hypothermia* (body temperature = 26°C). The diagnostic finding is the J wave, a positive wave interposed between the QRS and ST segment. It appears in all leads and, as the body temperature drops further, broadens and increases in size. The other changes are atrial fibrillation with bradycardia, ST depression and prolongation of the QT interval (QT_c = 0.65s).

B The electrocardiogram (2) shows inhibition of the ventricular pacemaker output in response to sensed myopotential signals (the patient was asked to push his hands together isometrically). This potential problem occurs with unipolar permanent pacemakers, i.e. a type of pacemaker in which only one wire travels to the heart. Electrons travel from the tip of this wire back to the anode, which is usually the wall of the pacemaker generator. Converting a unipolar pacemaker to bipolar will eliminate the myopotential sensing but requires a complete new pacemaker system. Many myopotential sensing problems can be minimized or eliminated through programming sensitivity to a lesser value (provided the sensing of intrinsic cardiac impulses is not adversely affected). Reprogramming the pacemaker to a fixed rate rather than demand mode may also be helpful.

C *Hyperkalaemia* (K^+ = 6.5mmol/L). The electrocardiogram (3) shows tall, pointed, narrow T waves in V_3–V_5. The P waves are broader and flatter than usual. As the serum potassium ion level increases further the R wave height will decrease, QRS complexes become wider and ST segment change occurs. Ventricular arrhythmias, atrioventricular block or asystole eventually occur (i.e. the changes are non-specific and can affect all parts of the electrocardiogram).

D *Pulmonary embolism.* The electrocardiogram (5) shows the so-called S_1, Q_3, T_3 pattern, bundle branch block and T inversion in the right precordial leads. However, these features develop in only a small minority of cases of pulmonary embolism (approximately 5%), i.e. a normal electrocardiograph tracing should never be held to refute a diagnosis of pulmonary embolism. The electrocardiogram returned to normal after pulmonary embolectomy when two large clots were removed.

E *Pericardial effusion.* The amplitude of the P, QRS and T waves is alternately high and low in consecutive beats. This is known as electrical alternans and is seen with a large pericardial effusion. Echocardiography is required to confirm the diagnosis.

F *Subarachnoid haemorrhage.* There is generalized extensive, deep, symmetrical T-wave inversion plus abnormal Q waves in the antero-lateral leads. This can be misdiagnosed as subendocardial infarction. Other electrocardiographic changes that occur with subarachnoid haemorrhage include: abnormally tall T waves, prominent U waves, ST segment elevation or depression, prolongation of the QT interval and arrhythmias (sinus tachycardia, sinus bradycardia, nodal rhythm, atrial fibrillation, ventricular tachycardia). A CT scan confirmed the diagnosis in this case.

Reference

Rowlands DJ. *Understanding the electrocardiogram.* Section 2: Morphological abnormalities. London: ICI plc, 1982.

Case 28

A case of chest pain following a recent pregnancy

History

A 29-year-old woman, whose health was excellent, began to experience episodes of substernal chest pain 6 days after the birth of her second child following an uncomplicated pregnancy and delivery. The pains persisted for 6 hours and the woman was admitted to hospital. No arteriosclerotic risk factors, including hypertension, smoking, diabetes, oral contraceptive use, family history of premature myocardial infarction or hyperlipoproteinaemia, were present. The electrocardiogram at admission is shown (1). The patient subsequently had an episode of ventricular fibrillation that responded to electric cardioversion. Coronary arteriography (2) was performed as an emergency procedure.

Questions

A What is the likely diagnosis in this case?
B What does the coronary arteriogram (2) show?
C What other causes of this abnormality do you know?
D What are the possible aetiological mechanisms for this presentation?
E How would you subsequently manage this patient?

Case 28

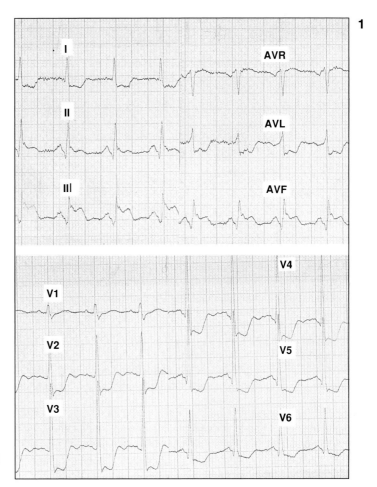

1 Electrocardiogram at admission.

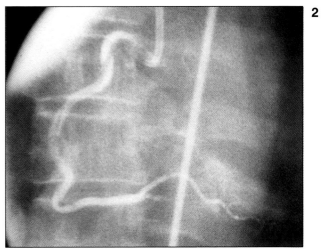

2 Coronary arteriogram.

Case 28

Answers

A The history and electrocardiogram (1) point to acute inferior (plus posterior [tall R wave V1–2]) myocardial infarction occurring in the postpartum period. This occurs mostly in primiparous women in their middle 20s, and usually within 1 to 2 weeks of delivery. Pre-eclampsia is an associated risk factor for its occurrence.

B The right coronary arteriogram (2) shows an extensive spiral dissection and the posterior descending branch is absent. The left coronary arteriogram (not shown) was entirely normal. Approximately one-third of all spontaneous primary coronary dissections described in women occur in the peripartum period. Presentation is with acute infarction, sudden death or unstable angina, with the left anterior descending artery affected more commonly than the right. The plane in which dissection develops is between the media and adventitia rather than intramedially, as in dissection of the aorta.

C Dissection also occurs within a coronary artery as a complication of procedures such as endarterectomy, insertion of vein grafts, cardiac catheterization, and angioplasty. No clear association with diseases that produce cystic medial necrosis in the aorta (such as Marfan's syndrome) has been established, however.

D Postpartum myocardial infarction is not necessarily related to atherosclerotic narrowing and can occur in normal coronary arteries. Coronary thrombo-embolism (possibly related to abnormalities of blood clotting associated with pregnancy), coronary arterial spasm (possibly related to the use of ergot alkaloids), as well as primary coronary arterial dissection, could all account for this clinical picture.

E Primary dissection of a coronary artery during pregnancy or the puerperium is frequently fatal. This patient survived an episode of primary ventricular fibrillation and was immediately given intravenous nitrates and opiates. The decision was taken not to perform emergency coronary bypass grafting, particularly as coronary flow was satisfactory. The patient's pain settled. Subsequent electrocardiograms showed a Q wave inferior infarction with a peak creatine kinase of 1500IU/l (normal 20–150IU/l). An exercise test performed six weeks after discharge showed no ischaemic abnormalities. Patients who develop dissection in the puerperium exhibit a risk of further such events in similar circumstances and this patient was, therefore, advised against future pregnancies.

References

Beary JF, Summer WR, Bulkley BH. Postpartum acute myocardial infarction: A rare occurrence of uncertain aetiology. *Am J Cardiol* 1979; 43:158-161.

Shaver PJ, Carrig TF, Baker WP. Postpartum coronary artery dissection. *Br Heart J* 1978; 40:83-86.

Postpartum collapse

History

A 24-year-old female collapsed suddenly 2 days after delivery of a normal male infant. She had complained of chest pains for a few hours before the episode, and a chest X-ray had been taken. Despite attempts at resuscitation, she died without regaining consciousness.

Question

A What is the differential diagnosis of sudden collapse in the early pueperium? What abnormality can you see on the chest X-ray (1)?

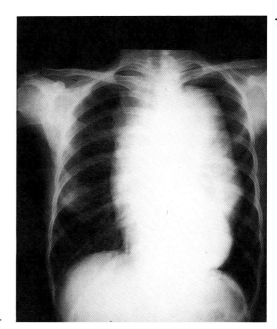

1 Posterior/anterior chest X-ray.

Answer

A You should consider obstetric causes (postpartum haemorrhage, septicaemia). Cardiovascular pathologies to consider are myocardial infarction, massive pulmonary embolism, and aortic dissection or rupture. In this patient a Type A aortic dissection had occurred. At postmortem examination there was evidence of cystic medial necrosis of the aortic wall.

Case 30

An important cause of hypoxaemia

History

A 58-year-old man presented with a 3-month history of progressive shortness of breath, fatigue and ankle swelling. There was no other relevant medical history. Examination revealed central cyanosis. The jugular venous pressure was markedly elevated. A right ventricular heave was felt over the precordium. Auscultation revealed a loud pulmonary component of the second heart sound and a soft systolic murmur. The lung fields were clear. The liver was enlarged 3cm below the costal margin. Blood gases breathing air revealed a PO_2 of 8kpa and PCO_2 of 4kpa. An electrocardiogram (1), chest radiograph (2) and echocardiogram (3) were performed.

Questions

A What does the electrocardiogram (1) show?
B What does the chest radiograph (2) show?
C What does the echocardiogram (3) show?
D What are the possible diagnoses in this case?
E What further investigations should be performed?

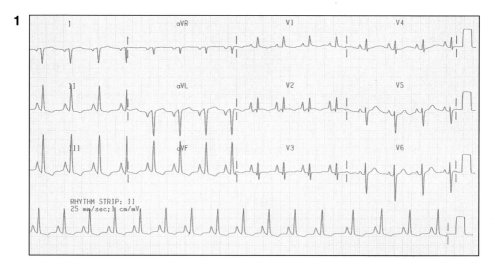

1

1 Electrocardiogram at presentation.

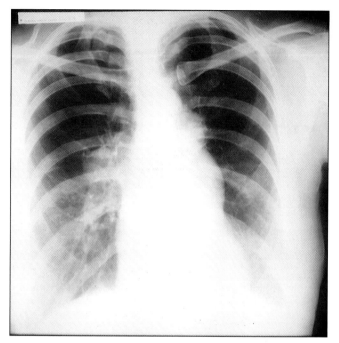

2 Chest radiograph at presentation.

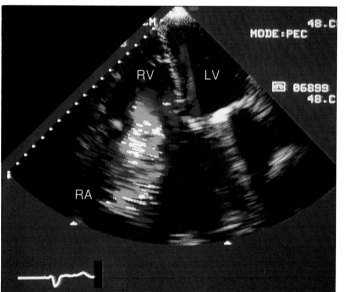

3 Cross-sectional echocardiogram (apical four-chamber view) with colour-flow imaging (frame in systole). LV, left ventricle; RA, right atrium; RV, right ventricle.

Case 30

Answers

A The electrocardiogram (**1**) shows right ventricular hypertrophy (criteria: a combined voltage of R in V_1 and S in V_6 of 10mm or more, an R wave taller than the S wave in V_1, an S wave deeper than the R wave in V_6, and right axis deviation). There is also evidence of P pulmonale, indicating right atrial hypertrophy.

B The chest radiograph (**2**) shows enlargement of the pulmonary arteries in the hila. There is also peripheral 'pruning' of the blood vessels associated with oligaemia. The findings are consistent with severe pulmonary hypertension.

C The cross-sectional echocardiogram with colour-flow imaging (**3**) is taken from the apical four-chamber view. There is dilatation of the right atrium and ventricle. The frame is taken in systole and shows a wide turbulent signal (blue and orange) filling the whole of the right atrium. The findings are consistent with severe tricuspid regurgitation. Continuous wave Doppler recording of the tricuspid regurgitant jet revealed a peak jet velocity of 4m/s, giving a calculated right ventricular/right atrial gradient of 64mmHg ($4 \times \text{velocity}^2$). The pulmonary artery systolic pressure is 64 + 10 (right atrial pressure) = 74mmHg (in absence of pulmonary stenosis).

D The investigations performed suggest severe pulmonary hypertension and the differential diagnosis is shown in **Table 1**. The most frequent causes are cor pulmonale, chronic thrombo-embolic pulmonary hypertension and primary pulmonary hypertension.

E A normal perfusion lung scan (using Technetium-99m) will exclude pulmonary embolism and the addition of a ventilation scan (obtained by inhalation of a radioactive gas such as krypton or xenon) increases the specificity of this technique. Pulmonary embolism usually produces a defect of perfusion but not of ventilation; most other conditions such as chronic obstructive airways disease and chest infections produce a perfusion defect and also impair ventilation, such that ventilation and perfusion are 'matched'. Pulmonary embolism can also produce matched defects, but in this situation the chest radiograph nearly always shows the infarct.

Lung function tests (spirometry, lung volumes, transfer factor) will usually differentiate those cases due to cor pulmonale. Right heart catheterization and pulmonary angiography is the 'gold standard' investigation for the diagnosis of pulmonary embolism (**4**), but it has disadvantages, the most important being its limited availability and a small but definite risk

- Cor pulmonale
- Chronic thrombo-embolic pulmonary hypertension
- Primary pulmonary hypertension
- Pulmonary veno-occlusive disease
- Eisenmenger's syndrome
- Left heart lesions, e.g. mitral valve disease
- Collagen vascular diseases
- Parasites (*Schistosoma*)
- Drug induced (aminorex and other appetite suppressants)

Table 1 Causes of severe pulmonary hypertension.

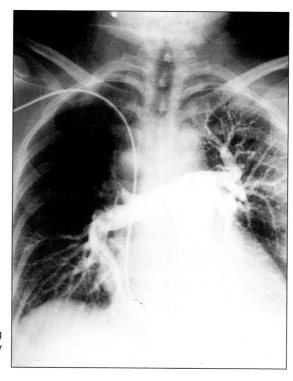

4 Pulmonary angiography showing perfusion defects due to pulmonary emboli in both lungs.

of mortality (especially in chronic thrombo-embolic pulmonary hypertension or primary pulmonary hypertension).

In this case pulmonary angiography showed multiple perfusion defects due to chronic thrombo-embolism and also confirmed the estimated pulmonary pressure. There were no obvious predisposing factors, i.e. no history of venous thrombosis and no evidence of neoplasia or clotting abnormalities.

The patient was given intravenous heparin by continuous infusion and warfarin was subsequently commenced. The natural history of chronic thrombo-embolic pulmonary hypertension is one of steady deterioration in most cases, with worsening heart failure. Death usually occurs within a few years of diagnosis. Occasionally, longer survival is seen and there are some cases reported showing recovery on long-term anticoagulation.

Reference

Hall RJC, Haworth SG. Disorders of the pulmonary circulation. In: *Diseases of the heart.* Julian DG, Camm AJ, Fox KM, Hall RJC, Poole-Wilson PA (eds). London: Baillière Tindall, 1989.

Case 31

A rare metabolic disease associated with coronary artery disease

History

A 35-year-old man presented with increasing angina of effort to his general practitioner and was referred to a local cardiologist for further investigations. The man had previously been diagnosed as hypertensive and was treated with nifedipine SR 10mg b.d. He was a life-long non-smoker. There was no family history of ischaemic heart disease but both his sisters had hypertension. On examination the blood pressure was 170/100mmHg. All pulses were present and no bruits were heard. There was clinical evidence of left ventricular hypertrophy. A number of blue-black telangiectases were noted on the lower trunk, buttocks and thighs (1 and 2). The patient said these had been present for a number of years. Fundal examination (3) revealed dilated and tortuous retinal vessels with aneurysmal dilatation of the small venules. Urinanalysis revealed proteinuria. Serum urea and electrolytes were normal. Fasting cholesterol was 4.7mmol/l and random blood sugar 5.0mmol/l. An electrocardiogram showed sinus rhythm, left ventricular hypertrophy and inverted T waves in the lateral chest leads.

Questions

A What further investigations of this patient's angina should be performed?
B What underlying condition is this patient suffering from and what other cardiovascular complications may occur?

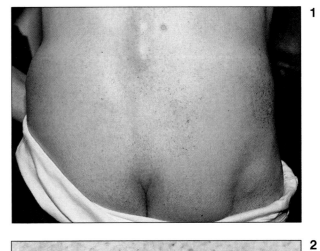

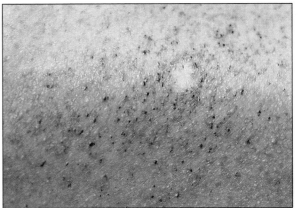

1 & 2 Skin appearance over the buttocks.

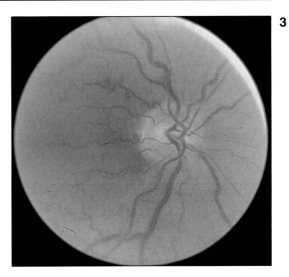

3 Dilated and tortuous retinal vessels with aneurysmal dilatation.

Case 31

Answers

A As angina is effort-related, a formal exercise test is useful as a provocative manoeuvre to induce myocardial ischaemia. The test is terminated either when the symptoms reported by the patient occur, when myocardial ischaemia has been detected, or at the patient's request. The electrocardiogram is used to detect acute myocardial ischaemia (defined as planar or down-sloping ST-segment depression or elevation of greater than 0.1mV, measured 80ms after the J point). It should be remembered that there are several causes of false-positive exercise electrocardiographic changes, including the presence of left ventricular hypertrophy, as in this case. In such circumstances stress testing associated with perfusion scintigraphy using thallium[201] provides greater overall sensitivity and specificity for diagnosing coronary artery disease. In this case the test was terminated after 5 minutes using a Bruce protocol due to the development of chest pain and dyspnoea associated with 0.2mV ST-segment depression in the antero-lateral leads.

The thallium images at peak exercise and following a 4-hour rest period are shown (4 and 5). The patient was treated with a larger dose of nifedipine and the addition of atenolol plus glyceryl trinitrate spray. Both angina and blood pressure control improved significantly. In view of his relatively young age, however, coronary arteriography was performed. This showed severe diffuse disease in the left anterior descending artery. The left circumflex and right coronary artery showed only minor narrowings, though.

B A dermatological opinion was obtained and this confirmed our suspicion that the telangiectases were angiokeratomas characteristic of Fabry's disease. A review of the patient's medical history revealed episodes of pain and paraesthesia in the extremities in adolescence but no diagnosis had previously been suggested. The patient also gave a history of intermittent nausea and abdominal pain.

Fabry's disease is an X-linked recessive disorder producing alpha-galactosidase A deficiency, leading to intracellular deposition of glycolipid in skin, kidneys, blood vessels and myocardium. The cardiovascular manifestations are variable due to accumulation in myocardium, conducting tissue, mitral/aortic valves and coronary arteries. Aortic stenosis, mitral insufficiency, dysrhythmias and angina pectoris can all occur. Renal hypertension may complicate the clinical picture. Left ventricular hypertrophy may be secondary to hypertension or primary due to storage cells containing glycolipids. Hence this patient has developed coronary artery disease consequent both to the underlying disease process and its hypertensive manifestations.

Reference

Becker AE, Schoorl R, Balk AG, *et al.* Cardiac manifestations of Fabry disease. *Am J Cardiol* 1975; **36**:829-835.

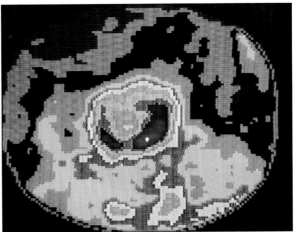

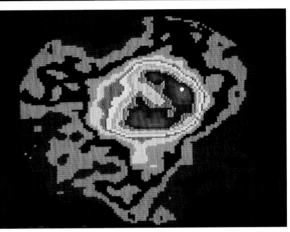

4 & 5 Thallium scan (**4**) at peak exercise (left anterior oblique view) showing impaired uptake in the anteroseptal region; (**5**) after 4 hours' rest there is complete redistribution (antero-posterior view) consistent with reversible ischaemia.

Case 32

An unusual cause of shortness of breath

History

A 65-year-old man with poor left ventricular function due to ischaemic cardiomyopathy complained of recurrent palpitations with associated slight dizziness. His drug treatment was frusemide 80mg once daily and lisinopril 5mg once daily. Clinical examination was unremarkable. A 24-hour Holter recording was performed and showed multifocal ventricular extrasystoles, couplets and frequent episodes of non-sustained ventricular tachycardia. He was commenced on antiarrhythmic therapy and the palpitations slowly improved. Six months later the patient experienced increasing breathlessness with a non-productive cough. On examination the pulse was 90 beats/min (regular); blood pressure 110/90mmHg lying and standing. The jugular venous pressure appeared normal. Auscultation revealed normal heart sounds but crepitations were heard at the lung bases. The patient's clinical appearance is shown in (1) and the chest radiographic appearance in (2).

Questions

A   What is the likely cause of the patient's present symptoms?
B   What further investigations should be performed in this case?
C   How would you subsequently manage this patient?

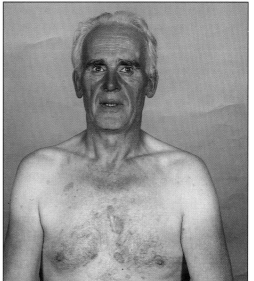

1 Clinical appearance of patient.

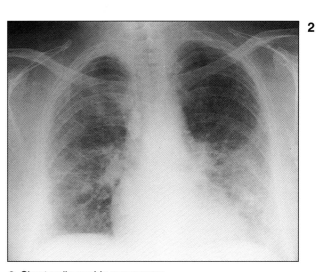

2 Chest radiographic appearance.

Case 32

Answers

A   While the patient's shortness of breath could have been due to progressive left ventricular dysfunction or the complication of a pulmonary embolus, the normal heart sounds and jugular venous pressure make either diagnosis less likely. The chest radiograph shows diffuse alveolar shadowing in both lung fields due to interstitial pneumonitis (the appearance is often mistaken for pulmonary oedema, particularly in patients known to have left ventricular dysfunction). The radiographic and clinical appearances (showing a photosensitive rash and facial slate-grey pigmentation) are consistent with adverse effects from amiodarone therapy. Both the slate-grey pigmentation and the pneumonitis are related to high-dose amiodarone intake and this patient had required 800mg daily for adequate control of his ventricular arrhythmia.

B   Pulmonary function tests should be performed. In this case, a restrictive lung defect was demonstrated (a small forced vital capacity [FVC], a reduced forced expiratory volume in one second [FEV$_1$] and a normal [FEV$_1$/FVC ratio], with a reduced total lung capacity and impaired transfer factor). Arterial blood gases should also be investigated – in this case they showed characteristic hypoxemia and hypocapnia.

C   Interstitial pneumonitis due to amiodarone therapy may lead to irreversible pulmonary fibrosis, although if the complication is recognised early enough withdrawal of amiodarone may produce regression. Treatment with corticosteroids may also be beneficial. In this case, however, amiodarone withdrawal resulted in resolution of symptoms and improvement in lung function over a 2-month period.

Alternative antiarrhythmic therapy was required and in view of the impaired left ventricular function the patient was commenced on mexiletine. This has been shown to have little effect on left ventricular ejection fraction even in patients with pre-existing left ventricular dysfunction. Satisfactory antiarrhythmic control was thus achieved.

Reference

Camm AJ. The recognition and management of tachyarrhythmias. In: *Diseases of the heart*. Julian DG, Camm AJ, Fox KM, Hall RJC, Poole-Wilson PA (eds). London: Baillière Tindall, 1989.

A 'classic' chest radiograph appearance

History

A 10-year-old boy attending a cardiology clinic was known to have an ejection systolic murmur audible at the left sternal edge and radiating to the pulmonary area. His electrocardiogram (1) and chest radiograph (2) are shown.

Questions

A What is the correct diagnosis of this patient's condition?
B What other physical signs may be present?
C What further investigations are appropriate in such a case?
D Comment on the management of this condition.

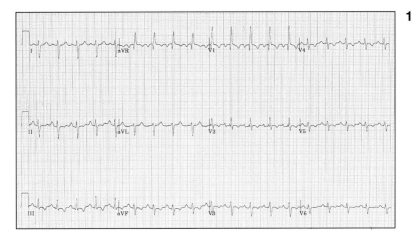

1

1 Electrocardiographic appearance.

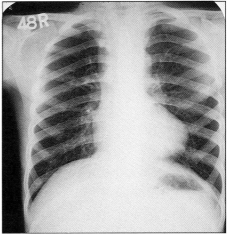

2

2 Chest radiograph appearance.

Case 33

Answers

A   The electrocardiogram (1) shows right axis deviation, right ventricular enlargement, and inverted T waves in the inferior and anterior leads. The chest radiograph shows a heart of normal size associated with diminished pulmonary vascularity. The heart shows a classic configuration of the 'coeur en sabot' ('like a wooden clog') due to right ventricular hypertrophy elevating its apex. This sign is generally seen in older patients with the tetralogy of Fallot. A right-sided aortic arch may sometimes also be present (though not in this particular patient).

B   Patients with tetralogy of Fallot develop central cyanosis and clubbing when there is a significant right-to-left shunt across the ventricular septal defect (VSD). In this case, a parasternal heave of right ventricular hypertrophy is present, and on auscultation a single second (aortic) sound is heard (due to pulmonary stenosis). The systolic murmur is due to pulmonary stenosis, not the VSD.

C   Cross-sectional echocardiography (3) is diagnostic (particularly using the subcostal view to obtain oblique views of the right ventricular outflow tract). Magnetic resonance imaging (MRI), if available, also clearly demonstrates the severity of subpulmonary obstruction and the precise nature of the VSD. Cardiac catheterization and angiocardiography are still needed for full documentation of the pulmonary arterial pathways, however.

D   All patients with the tetralogy should have a totally corrective operation, but the timing of this is often a matter of debate. Palliative surgery in the form of a shunt operation will ameliorate cyanosis (which impairs growth and intellectual development) but will not prevent strokes or brain abscess, which can complicate the condition. In most centres, a shunt operation (Blalock–Taussig – subclavian artery to pulmonary artery; Waterston – ascending aorta to pulmonary artery) is initially performed to palliate symptomatic infants and the definitive operation undertaken when the child is older (age 5–10 years).

Reference

Tynan M, Anderson RH. Congenital heart disease. In: *Diseases of the heart.* Julian DG, Camm AJ, Fox KM, Hall RJC, Poole-Wilson PA (eds). London: Baillière Tindall, 1989.

3

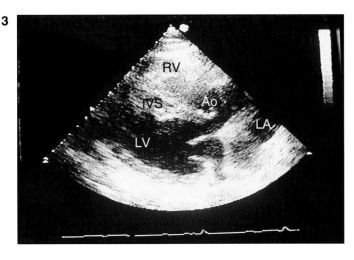

3 Two-dimensional echo-cardiogram (parasternal long-axis view) of patient with tetralogy of Fallot. Overriding of the aorta (Ao) is present, together with dropout of echoes between the interventricular septum and aorta. RV, right ventricle; LV, left ventricle; LA, left atrium; IVS, interventricular septum.

A case of post-myocardial infarction angina

History

A 50-year-old man presented with frequent angina of effort following a myocardial infarction two months previously (confirmed at the time by a fourfold rise in creatine kinase). The electrocardiogram now showed sinus rhythm and left bundle branch block with inverted T waves in the antero-septal leads. The patient continued to experience angina despite treatment with atenolol and isosorbide mononitrate and an exercise thallium[201] scan was therefore arranged (1 and 2), followed by cardiac catheterization and coronary arteriography.

Questions

A What does the thallium scan show?
B What do the coronary angiograms (3 and 4) show?
C Comment on the further management of this patient's angina.

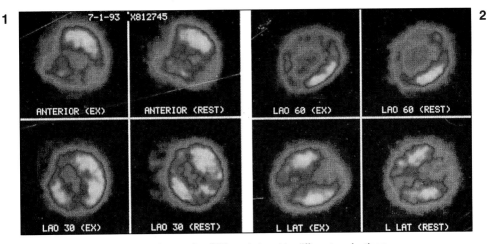

1 & 2 Thallium images at peak exercise (EX) and at rest in different projections.

Case 34

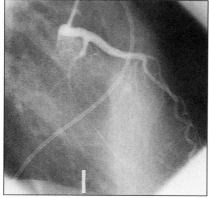

3 Coronary angiogram (right anterior oblique view).

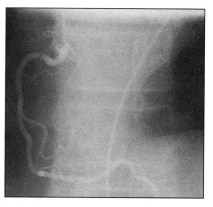

4 Right coronary angiogram (left anterior oblique view).

Answers

A Exercise testing in patients with post-infarction angina is performed for risk stratification and to assess the severity and prognostic importance of the coronary artery lesions. Certain electrocardiographic features, which include the presence of left bundle branch block, render the test difficult to interpret. In this situation a thallium (Tl) exercise test is quite useful as it does not depend on exercise-induced ST-segment changes. The uptake of thallium into the myocardium depends on the integrity of the Na^+–K^+ ATPase pump on its surface membrane. When maximum predicted heart rate is achieved during the exercise test, or when there is chest pain sufficient to terminate exercise, 80MBq of Tl^{201} is injected intravenously. Imaging is commenced 5 minutes later, usually using 3 different projections (left anterior oblique [LAO], anterior [AP] and left lateral).

This patient's thallium planar scan suggests the presence of ischaemia ('a cold spot') at peak exercise, affecting the inferoapical region of the myocardium, as seen on AP and LAO 60° projections. There is incomplete redistribution of activity after 4 hours of rest. The picture thus suggests the presence of reversible ischaemia, probably affecting the circumflex and/or right coronary artery.

B The left coronary angiogram (**3**) shows a proximal occlusion of the circumflex branch while the left anterior descending branch appears normal. The right coronary angiogram (**4**) shows only minor irregularity of the vessel wall. A left ventricular angiogram was also performed (not shown), and this revealed preserved left ventricular function with no evidence of a significant myocardial infarction.

C   Post-infarction angina, particularly if resistant to medical therapy, is a clinical situation in which cardiac surgery is possible but associated with an increased risk. In the presence of single vessel disease and preserved left ventricular function, experience has shown that coronary angioplasty (PTCA) is often effective in restoring coronary flow and abolishing symptoms. Acute complications and late restenosis are more common following PTCA in this situation compared to stable angina, however. In this case PTCA was successfully performed. Using a Judkins guiding catheter positioned in the left coronary ostia, a high torque 'floppy' radio-opaque steerable guide wire was negotiated through the circumflex occlusion. A 3mm diameter 'monorail' balloon catheter was then placed over the guide wire and through the occlusion. Once the balloon was across the lesion 2 dilations, each of 60 seconds' duration and each at an inflation pressure of 6 atmospheres, were performed (5). This resulted in complete restoration of blood flow to the distal circumflex artery with a normal lumen at the site of inflations (6). The patient's angina settled and anti-anginal therapy was successfully reduced over the next few months.

5

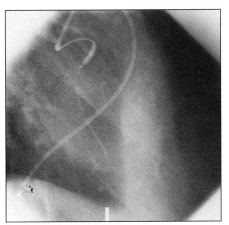

6

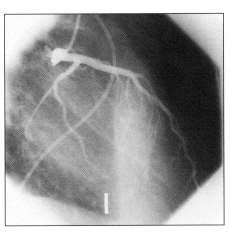

5 PTCA to circumflex occlusion, showing the radio-opaque guide wire in the distal vessel and the balloon catheter inflated.

6   Left coronary angiogram (right anterior oblique view) following successful angioplasty.

Reference

Shiu, MF. Interventional Cardiac Catheterization: Transluminal angioplasty. In: *Diseases of the heart*. Julian DG, Camm AJ, Fox KM, Hall RJC, Poole-Wilson PA (eds). London: Baillière Tindall, 1989.

Case 35

Palpitations in an otherwise well young man

History

A 24-year-old man with a 6-month history of intermittent palpitations associated with slight dizziness was referred to a cardiology clinic by his general practitioner. There was no other relevant history. Clinical examination was entirely normal. The patient actually experienced his symptoms during routine electrocardiography.

Questions

A   What do the electrocardiograms (1 and 2) show?
B   What further investigations should be performed?
C   What treatment would you recommend for this patient?

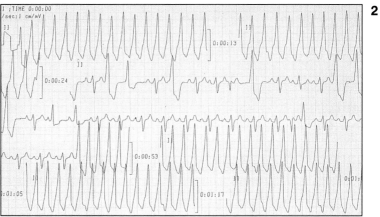

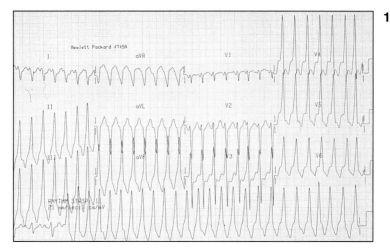

1 & 2 Electrocardiographic appearance.

Case 35

Answers

A The electrocardiograms (**1** and **2**) show a repetitive monomorphic broad complex tachycardia. The QRS complex is 160ms wide, slightly irregular in rate, with a left bundle branch block morphology and an inferior axis. Furthermore, there is atrioventricular dissociation as seen in leads AVR and V6. These features are consistent with ventricular tachycardia originating from the right ventricular outflow tract (RVOT). Such tachycardias are usually non-sustained and present as sinus rhythm interrupted by repetitive monomorphic ventricular extrasystoles or salvos of ventricular tachycardia.

B Patients with 'idiopathic' monomorphic ventricular tachycardia require careful assessment of the right ventricle to exclude subclinical cardiomyopathy. Two-dimensional echocardiography should be performed, and right ventricular angiography plus endomyocardial biopsy should also both be considered. Exercise testing can precipitate or suppress such tachycardias and may be useful in evaluating the effects of drug treatment, etc. Programmed electrical stimulation is performed in most patients with recurrent 'idiopathic' tachycardias to evaluate possible therapeutic options. However, RVOT is not usually induced by this means.

C The principal mechanism of many ventricular tachycardias is re-entry movement. Other important mechanisms are reflection (a form of micro-entry), triggered or abnormal automaticity and macrore-entry around the His–Purkinje system. RVOT tachycardia is thought to originate through abnormal automaticity or triggered activity and is induced by intracellular calcium overload. Hence, verapamil is often useful in this condition, although beta-blockers and Vaughan Williams class I antiarrhythymic agents can also be effective.

References

Buxton AE, Marchlinski FE, Doherty JU, *et al.* Repetitive, monomorphic ventricular tachycardia: clinical and electrophysiologic characteristics in patients with and patients without heart disease. *Am. J. Cardiol.* 1984; 54:997-1002.

Coumel P. Repetitive monomorphic ventricular tachycardia. In: *Cardiac Pacing and Electrophysiology.* 3rd Edn. WB Saunders Company, 1991.

A case demonstrating the value of early coronary angiography for persistent angina

History

A 38-year-old man was referred to a cardiology clinic with angina following a myocardial infarction 3 months previously. The patient had initially received intravenous streptokinase for acute myocardial infarction and had been taking oral aspirin and atenolol since discharge. He was intolerant of oral nitrate preparations (producing severe headache). Clinical examination was unremarkable. The electrocardiogram at time of clinic consultation is shown in (1). The patient underwent coronary arteriography within the next few days.

Questions

A   What does the electrocardiogram (1) show?
B   What do the coronary angiograms (2 and 3) show?
C   How would you manage this patient's symptoms?

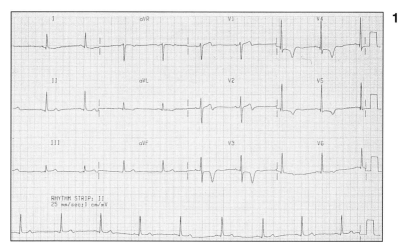 **1**

1 Electrocardiographic appearance.

Case 36

2

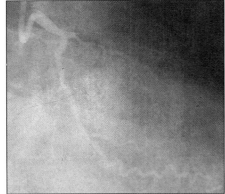

2 Left coronary angiogram.

3

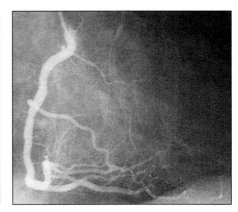

3 Right coronary angiogram.

Answers

A The electrocardiogram (1) shows evidence of a non-Q-wave anterior myocardial infarction, with marked T-wave inversion in leads V_{3-6} plus I and AVL. Although the initial (in-hospital) mortality of such cases is low, the longer-term prognosis seems to be at least as bad as that for Q-wave (or 'transmural') infarction. Furthermore, the incidence of unstable angina and Q-wave infarction in the first year is up to 46% and 21%, respectively. In the presence of angina in such a patient early coronary angiography is mandatory, therefore.

B (2) shows the left coronary angiogram (right anterior oblique view with caudal tilt). There is a normal left main stem and normal circumflex vessel (with a large obtuse marginal branch). The left anterior descending artery is occluded very proximally, however. Despite this, the patient's left ventricular function was very well preserved with no major regional wall motion abnormalities demonstrated by left ventricular angiography (not shown here) at time of cardiac catheterization. This would clearly account for the electrocardiographic changes. (3) shows the right coronary artery (right anterior oblique view), which is normal, but which exhibits a marked retrograde filling of the left anterior descending artery (to the right of the illustration) via collateral vessels, reaching back to the first septal branch.

Case 36

C A total vessel occlusion, as seen here, that is well collateralized is functionally equivalent to a 90% stenosis. In this situation the myocardium remains viable, but results in clinically apparent ischaemia during periods of increased oxygen demand. This in turn results in effort angina, though usually not truly unstable angina. The possibility of surgical intervention should be discussed in such a case as the symptoms are limiting enough to warrant bypass surgery. A percutaneous recanalization attempt (PTCA) is far less costly and invasive, however. This should be considered as a prime option in many such cases, therefore, with surgery being reserved should angioplasty prove impossible. Furthermore, although technical success of a surgical intervention is virtually guaranteed in a case of single vessel disease it is no more likely than angioplasty to increase longevity.

In this particular case coronary angioplasty was successful in abolishing the patient's symptoms. Using a 8F Amplatz guiding catheter, a high torque steerable 'floppy' guide wire crossed the occlusion with the aid of a deflated monorail 3mm diameter balloon catheter for support. The balloon was then advanced and inflated (4) at the site of occlusion. This resulted in successful recanalization of the left anterior descending artery (5) and complete disappearance of the collaterals from the right coronary artery. The duration and the total length of the occlusion were both relatively short in this case, providing a good chance of success. Longer length occlusions and those present for over 6 months are much less likely to result in successful recanalization with angioplasty, however.

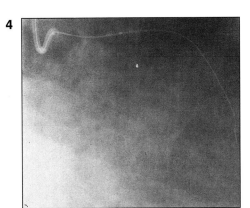

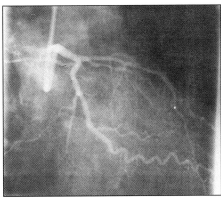

4 PTCA procedure, showing guide wire positioned at distal part of left anterior descending artery with balloon catheter inflated at site of occlusion.

5 Successful recanalization of left anterior descending artery.

Case 37

Patients presenting with tachycardias

Question

What does the electrocardiogram show and what treatment would you recommend in each of the following cases?

A Patient A presented to the cardiology clinic with palpitations. He was known to suffer from angina pectoris (1).

B Patient B presented to the casualty department having suffered palpitations for the previous 4 hours. He had previously experienced similar attacks of shorter duration but was receiving no regular treatment (2).

C Patient C, a 30-year-old nursing sister, presented with palpitations whose sudden onset had occurred while she had been on duty in the coronary care unit (3).

D Patient D, 50 years of age, was known to suffer from mitral valve prolapse, and routine electrocardiography was performed. She was asymptomatic and was on no regular medication (4).

E Patient E, a 60-year-old man who suffered from chronic airways disease, presented with palpitations and pre-syncope (5).

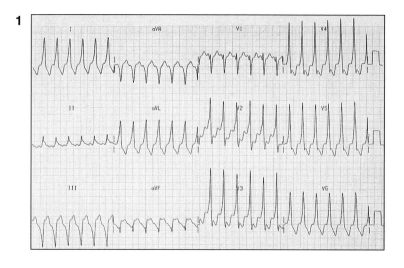

2

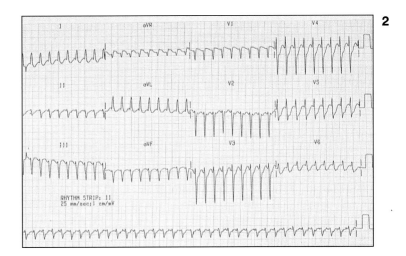

3

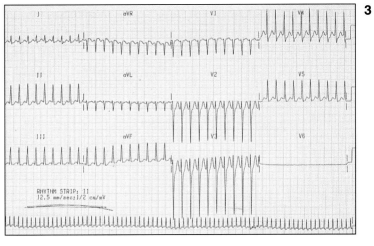

4

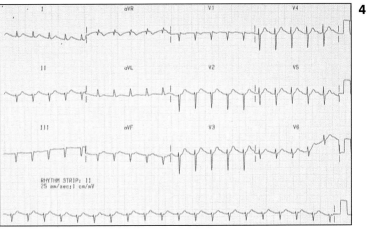

Case 37

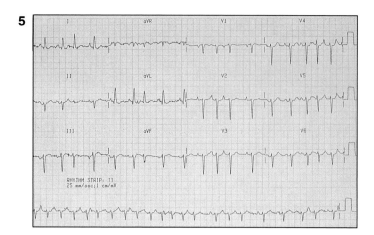

Answers

A (1) shows a broad complex tachycardia (rate 160 beats/min) with a left bundle branch block pattern. Tachycardias with broad ventricular complexes are due to ventricular tachycardia or supraventricular tachycardia – the latter either with bundle branch block during sinus rhythm or with rate-related bundle branch block (i.e. phasic aberrant intraventricular conduction). When the QRS complex is predominantly negative in lead V_1 (left bundle branch block pattern), differentiating between ventricular and supraventricular tachycardia can sometimes be difficult, particularly if a 12 lead electrocardiogram during sinus rhythm is not available. In this patient, however, there is clear evidence of atrioventricular association (lead II and V_1) consistent with an atrial tachycardia with 1:1 atrioventricular conduction and a bundle branch block pattern (the bundle branch block was also present in sinus rhythm). Most atrial tachycardias with atrial rates in the region of 180–200 or less will usually be associated with 1:1 AV conduction (unless AV nodal function is depressed by drugs or disease). More rapid atrial rates will normally show 2:1 AV block.

The first treatment approach should be vagal stimulation and carotid sinus massage is the form usually employed. If vagal stimulation does not work intravenous verapamil should be tried. Other drugs, such as digoxin and flecainide may also be effective. If drugs are ineffective or if the patient's clinical condition necessitates an early return to sinus rhythm, synchronized DC cardioversion should be carried out. If prophyaxis against recurrence is required beta-blockers, digoxin, verapamil, disopyramide or flecainide are effective in individual patients usually through a process of trial and error regarding effectiveness and tolerability.

B Figure 2 shows a narrow complex regular tachycardia at a rate of 230 beats/minute. Atrial complexes are seen immediately before and also immediately after each QRS complex (e.g. lead I and V_5) and the P-P rate is approximately 300 beats/minute. These appearances are consistent with atrial flutter with (AV) block. Carotid sinus massage will increase the degree of AV block temporarily and this can be useful in diagnosis of the rhythm, as the typical saw-tooth pattern becomes more obvious(especially in leads II and Vl). The ventricular rate is usually an integral sub-division of the atrial rate (e.g. 2:1 AV block producing a ventricular rate of 150) but this was not the case in this patient.

The aims of treatment are, first, to control the ventricular rate, and secondly to restore and maintain sinus rhythm. Intravenous verapamil will slow the ventricular rate by increasing atrioventricular block. In the presence of an isolated event or when urgent treatment is required, low energy DC cardioversion is frequently effective in restoring sinus rhythm. If flutter cannot be cardioverted or if it frequently recurs digoxin may be helpful in inducing atrial fibrillation, which may then have a controlled ventricular rate. The combination of digoxin and quinidine or disopyramide may result in restoration of sinus rhythm. These drugs are also useful in the treatment of chronic prophylaxis, and thus clearly required in this case in view of the patient's recurrent symptoms.

C (3) shows another narrow complex regular tachycardia (rate 250 beats/minute). No P waves are clearly identified. This is an example of a junctional tachycardia with the re-entrant pathway entirely within the AV node (i.e. atrioventricular nodal re-entrant tachycardia [AVNRT]). Initiation is by an atrial premature beat which enters the AV node, travels antegradely down a slow pathway to depolarize the ventricles, and then passes retrogradely up a fast conducting pathway to depolarize the atrial myocardium and thus complete the reentrant loop. This is a 'slow-fast' form of AVNRT and the retrograde P wave is usually hidden in the QRS complex or occurs immediately afterwards.

Acute termination of AVNRT can be performed by vagotonic manoeuvres or by intravenous injection of verapamil or adenosine. Long-term control is usually achieved using drugs which prolong the refractoriness of the AV node (e.g. verapamil or beta-blockers).

D (4) shows another narrow complex regular tachycardia, the ventricular rate being 120 beats/minute. The QRS complexes appear to occur before any P waves, which suggests a junctional tachycardia (non-paroxysmal type). In this patient the P waves are not really visible, suggesting they may be buried in the QRS complex. Alternatively, there may be failure to conduct retrogradely so that the atria may not depolarize at all. Non-paroxysmal AV junctional tachycardia is due to accelerated automatic discharge from the AV junctional zone and is usually gradual in onset. The patient had no symptoms and so no antiarrhythmic therapy was thought necessary.

E Figure 5 shows rapid irregular discrete P waves of different morphologies and an irregular rate narrow QRS complex. This suggests a diagnosis of multifocal atrial tachycardia, which is a relatively rare arrhythmia. It is seen in association with lung disease, digitalis toxicity, and diabetes. If it occurs in a patient receiving digitalis, treatment requires stopping digitalis and giving potassium replacement if the serum potassium is not abnormally elevated. In a patient not receiving digitalis, the underlying cause should be treated. The use of digitalis in combination with a calcium antagonist (or a beta-blocker, if not contraindicated) may be useful in slowing the ventricular rate. Conversion to sinus rhythm (by cardioversion, or by drugs – e.g. quinidine) is not usually successful, neither is the long-term prevention of recurrence (using drugs that stabilize the atrial myocardium, e.g. quinidine, disopyramide, procainamide).

Reference

Camm AJ. The recognition and management of tachyarrhythmias. In: *Diseases of the heart.* Julian DG, Camm AJ, Fox KM, Hall RJC, Poole-Wilson PA (eds). London: Baillière Tindall, 1989.

Case 38

A young man with cardiomegaly

History

A 25-year-old man presented with a 2-month history of increasing fatigue and breathlessness. He had also recently noticed some mild ankle swelling. Clinical examination revealed a pulse of 110 beats/minute, which was regular and of small volume. The jugular venous pressure was markedly elevated. A gallop rhythm and a soft pan-systolic murmur were heard on auscultation. An electrocardiogram (1) showed first degree atrioventricular block and left ventricular hypertrophy. A chest radiograph revealed cardiomegaly and pulmonary venous congestion. Echocardiography with Doppler examination was performed (2 and 3).

Questions

A What do the echocardiogram (1) and Doppler examination (2 and 3) show and what further information should be derived from the Doppler results?
B What further investigations should be performed to aid the management of this patient?
C Comment on the treatment regimen of such a case.

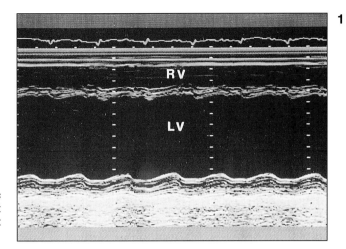

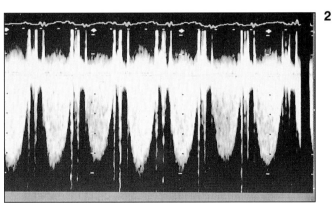

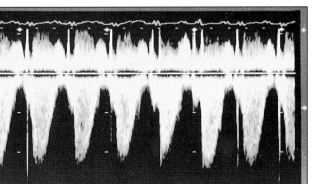

1 Echocardiographic appearance. RV, right ventricle; LV, left ventricle.

2 & 3 Doppler recordings from the mitral (**2**) and tricuspid (**3**) valves obtained from the cardiac apex (each division on the vertical line is 1m/sec).

Case 38

Answers

A The M-mode echocardiogram (1) shows that the left ventricular end-diastolic dimension (measured from the R wave of the electrocardiogram) is greatly enlarged (8cm). The end-systolic dimension is also much greater than normal so that the change between diastole and systole (percentage fractional shortening) is small. These features are consistent with a diagnosis of dilated cardiomyopathy and the potential aetiology is shown in **Table 1**. The right ventricular dimensions are normal but this is not always the case in this condition.

(2) shows a continuous wave Doppler spectral trace, obtained from the apex of the heart, which demonstrates the presence of mitral regurgitation. The regurgitant jet is seen as a high-velocity systolic signal flowing away from the transducer (i.e. below the zero line), the peak velocity of the curve being 5m/sec. Forward flow through the mitral valve is shown above the baseline (towards the transducer) and this is usually of a much lower velocity. Unfortunately, the velocity of flow within the regurgitant jet is not helpful in assessing the severity of mitral incompetence and account must be taken of other factors, including left atrial size and left ventricular function. Both pulsed and colour flow Doppler mapping may be helpful in assessing the severity of incompetence, but again the results must be interpreted with caution. Using pulsed Doppler in this case, the regurgitant jet was detected mainly near the mitral leaflets, and in view of the poor ventricular function was therefore thought to reflect mild ('functional') mitral regurgitation.

(3) shows another continuous wave spectral trace (velocity of 2m/sec only), demonstrating the additional presence of tricuspid regurgitation. When the peak velocity is <2.5m/sec, the regurgitation is likely to be 'physiological' rather than pathological. However, if a complete velocity envelope is not obtained, uncertainty may exist as to the precise peak systolic velocity. In this situation pulsed and colour Doppler may again be helpful in determining the severity of incompetence. The peak velocity also offers the opportunity of measuring the systolic gradient between the right ventricle and right atrium (gradient = $4 \times$ [peak velocity]^2). Using an arbitrary value of 10mmHg for the right atrial pressure the peak right ventricular pressure (gradient + 10mmHg) can be estimated. If there is no pulmonary stenosis then the pulmonary artery systolic pressure will, therefore, be the same (in this case, approximately 30mmHg).

• Idiopathic (conditioning – factors such as hypertension, alcohol, pregnancy may be evident)
• Infections
• Drugs (toxicity, hypersensitivity)
• Metabolic problems
• Deficiency states
• Collagen diseases
• Endocrine disorders (e.g. thyrotoxicosis)
• Muscular dystrophies (family history?).

Table 1 Aetiology of dilated cardiomyopathy.

B   Before making a confident diagnosis of dilated cardiomyopathy (**Table 1**), pre-existing coronary artery disease, valvular heart disease, hypertension, etc., should all be excluded. Cardiac catheterization and coronary arteriography often provide important information to this end. The left ventricular filling (end-diastolic) pressure and the pulmonary artery/capillary wedge pressures should be measured during this procedure. The latter allow calculation of the transpulmonary gradient (mean pulmonary artery [PA] - mean pulmonary wedge pressure [PAW]), which is important if cardiac transplantation is being considered. Irreversible pulmonary hypertension remains a contraindication to orthotopic cardiac transplantation and pulmonary vasodilator therapy (using intravenous sodium nitroprusside, for example) should be employed at the time of catheterization in an attempt to assess reversibility of elevated pulmonary vascular resistance:

$$\text{pulmonary vascular resistance} = \frac{\text{PA - PAW}}{\text{cardiac output}}\text{; normal range} < 2.5 \text{ units}$$

Although there are no specific histological findings in dilated cardiomyopathy an endomyocardial biopsy may occasionally be useful in excluding particular heart muscle diseases, including myocarditis. Ambulatory Holter monitoring to look for complex ventricular beats and non-sustained ventricular tachycardia (increased incidence in dilated cardiomyopathy) provides prognostic information in patients with idiopathic dilated cardiomyopathy. It will also assess the need for antiarrhythmic therapy. Radionuclide imaging (using $^{99}TC^M$ gated ventriculography) will provide further information on left ventricular function (e.g. ejection fraction), the results being comparable to those obtained using contrast angiography.

C   The basic treatment of dilated cardiomyopathy is mainly pharmacological. Diuretics are the mainstay, loop diuretics such as frusemide being most commonly used. Angiotensin-converting enzyme (Ace) inhibitors will produce significant symtomatic and haemodynamic improvement at rest and during exercise. Several studies have now also shown that Ace inhibitors will reduce mortality and progression of the disease process in all grades of heart failure. Digoxin may play a small role in the case of sinus rhythm, while its role in a patient with associated atrial fibrillation is well established. Antiarrhythmic agents (e.g. mexiletene or amiodarone) may prove useful in patients with higher grade ventricular arrhythmias. Anticoagulation with warfarin is useful in preventing or treating venous thrombosis and may also be helpful in the treatment of patients with echocardiographic evidence of mural thrombus.

Cardiac transplantation provides the best chance of long-term survival in suitable patients, and also offers a severe heart failure with substantial improvement in the quality of life. Transplantation centres vary in their top age limit for accepting cases, but between 50 and 60 years is the norm. It is important that the patient is referred early before the development of renal failure, pulmonary embolism, recurrent chest infections and cardiac cachexia, all of which greatly influence operative risk and post-operative survival.

Reference

Littler WA. Dilated cardiomyopathy. In: *Diseases of the heart.* Julian DG, Camm AJ, Fox KM, Hall RJC, Poole-Wilson PA. (eds). London: Baillière Tindall, 1989.

Case 39

Echocardiography in a patient with a heart murmur

History

A 30-year-old woman was referred to a cardiology clinic because her general practitioner had noticed a heart murmur. She had no symptoms and was previously unaware of the condition. Following clinical examination echocardiography (1 and 2) was performed.

Questions

A   What do the echocardiograms (1 and 2) show?
B   What further investigations may be useful in such a patient?
C   Comment on the management of this patient.

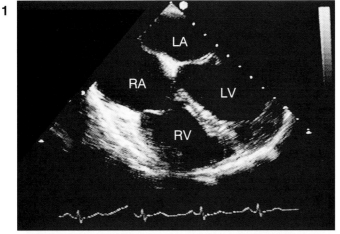

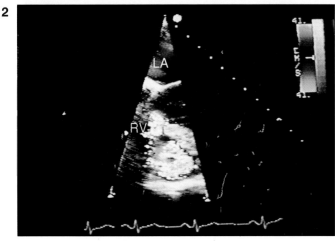

1 & 2 Echocardiographic appearance. RA, right atrium; LA, left atrium; RV, right ventricle; LV, left ventricle.

Answers

A (1) shows a ventricular septal defect using cross-sectional echocardiography (subcostal approach). (2) combines part of this image with colour flow Doppler mapping to show a left-to-right shunt through the septal defect. Cross-sectional echocardiography is the investigation of choice in this condition and can distinguish between the different types of septal defect that occur (perimembranous, supracristal or muscular). Furthermore, both pulsed and colour flow Doppler echocardiography will demonstrate the intracardiac shunt and can also indirectly assess the pulmonary artery pressure.

B Cardiac catheterization is generally no longer needed for diagnosis of a ventricular septal defect but can provide additional useful information. The right heart catheter usually follows the normal course to the pulmonary trunk but sometimes the defect may be crossed by the catheter, and the left ventricle and aorta may be entered from the right ventricle. There is a step up in oxygen saturation in the right ventricle, which is extremely useful in quantitating the left to right shunt (**Appendix 1**). Right ventricular and pulmonary arterial systolic pressures should be measured: the results will depend on the size of the defect and the pulmonary vascular resistance. The right atrial, left ventricular and aortic pressures are usually normal. Left ventricular contrast angiography in the left anterior oblique view allows localization of the septal defect (3).

C The majority of patients with a ventricular septal defect in adulthood require no specific treatment. Patients who, for one reason or another, have not been diagnosed in infancy should be considered for cardiac catheterization and corrective surgery when they have signs of high pulmonary blood flow, cardiomegaly or congestive cardiac failure. All patients with a ventricular septal defect need antibiotic prophylaxis against bacterial endocarditis.

Reference

Tynan M, Anderson RH. Congenital heart disease. In: *Diseases of the heart*. Julian DG, Camm AJ, Fox KM, Hall RJC, Poole-Wilson PA (eds). London: Baillière Tindall, 1989.

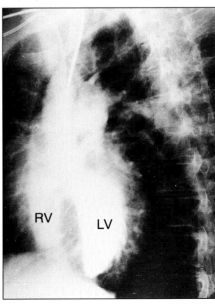

3

3 Left ventricular angiography (left anterior oblique view) demonstrating a perimembranous ventricular septal defect. LV, left ventricle; RV, right ventricle.

Case 39

Appendix: Shunt detection by oximetry

The ratio of pulmonary to systemic flow is estimated, i.e.

$$\frac{\text{Pulmonary}}{\text{Systemic flow}} = \frac{\text{Arterial saturation} - \text{mixed venous saturation \%}}{\text{Pulmonary venous} - \text{pulmonary artery saturation \%}}$$

98% is substituted for pulmonary venous saturation as pulmonary vein sampling is not possible unless there is an atrial septal defect or trans-septal catheterization is performed.

Mixed venous saturation is calculated as:

$$\frac{(3 \times \text{superior vena cava saturation}) + (1 \times \text{inferior vena cava saturation})}{4}$$

A simplified saturation run during catheterization involves sampling from:

Superior vena cava
High right atrium
Mid right atrium
Low right atrium
Inferior vena cava

Right ventricle
Main pulmonary artery
Aorta

An important cause of angina

History

A 50-year-old man presented with a 6-month history of angina of effort with associated breathlessness. A systolic murmur was heard all over the praecordium and an echocardiogram (1) was requested. The patient subsequently underwent cardiac catheterization (3).

Questions

A   Comment on the echocardiographic appearance (1).
B   What else should echocardiography provide in this case?
C   What information would be required from cardiac catheterization in this patient?

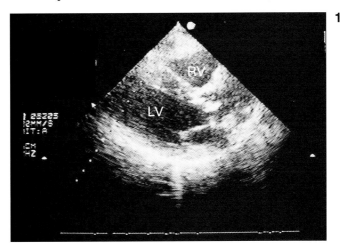

1 Echocardiographic appearance. RV, right ventricle; LV, left ventricle.

Case 40

Answers

A A cross-sectional image from the parasternal long-axis view is shown in (**1**). The aortic leaflets are markedly calcific with probable reduced separation ability. The interventricular septum shows marked hypertrophy (the posterior ventricular wall is not so well visualized) and there is dilatation of the aortic root. The findings are consistent with a diagnosis of significant aortic stenosis with post-stenotic dilatation of the ascending aorta.

B Assessment of the degree of aortic stenosis from the echocardiogram alone is frequently unreliable unless the lesion is very severe (as in this case) or very mild and a Doppler echocardiogram is therefore required in such a case. Using the modified Bernoulli equation ($P = 4V^2$, where P = pressure gradient [mmHg] and V = peak velocity at a narrowing [in m/sec]), the peak pressure difference across the aortic valve is calculated by continuous wave Doppler. This method is very reliable, widely used, and has replaced the need for cardiac catheterization to obtain the aortic valve gradient in many centres. It should be noted, however, that this is an instantaneous gradient (**2**) and not the same as the 'peak to peak' pressure difference recorded at catheterization (**3**); the peak pressure difference is usually higher and occurs earlier.

While an electrocardiogram and chest radiograph may reveal evidence of left ventricular enlargement, echocardiography should also be used to evaluate the left ventricular size and its ability to contract. When aortic stenosis is very advanced and heart failure develops, left ventricular wall motion is decreased and this is assessed as a reduction in percentage fractional shortening. In some patients, considerable left ventricular dilatation also occurs at this stage, although left ventricular wall thickness remains increased. In other patients there is only a slight increase in left ventricular dimensions, but wall movement is poor.

C As such good information about the aortic valve gradient and left ventricular function can now be obtained non-invasively, cardiac catheterization is often needed only to assess the state of the coronary arteries. Aortography should be performed, however, as it allows concomitant aortic regurgitation to be assessed. In this case the aortic valve was also crossed retrogradely and a peak-to-peak (left ventricle vs aorta) systolic gradient was obtained. In general, gradients > 50mmHg indicate significant aortic stenosis if cardiac output is normal. The coronary arteries were normal in this patient and he was subsequently referred for elective aortic valve replacement.

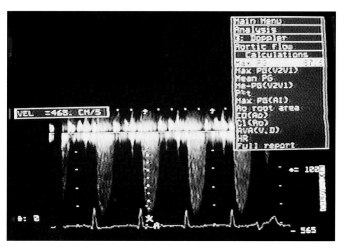

2 Continuous wave Döppler recording of the velocity of blood flow in the aortic root (obtained from the cardiac apex). The peak velocity is 4.7 m/sec, corresponding to a transvalvar gradient of approximately 90mmHg. Each division on the vertical line is 1 m/sec.

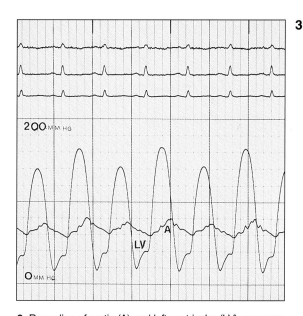

3 Recording of aortic (A) and left ventricular (LV) pressures obtained at cardiac catheterization (0–200mmHg range). The peak-to-peak gradient varies due to the presence of left ventricular alternans. This is the result of alteration in force of contraction of cardiac muscle and indicates severe disease. The aortic pulse tracing is also very slow rising (i.e. anacrotic).

123

Case 41

Shortness of breath following a myocardial infarction

History

A 50-year-old man who suffered an extensive myocardial infarction became suddenly short of breath in the following week. Echocardiography (1 and 2) was arranged to assess global left ventricular function.

Questions

A   What do the echocardiograms (1 and 2) show?
B   What further investigations may be appropriate and what treatment would you recommend?

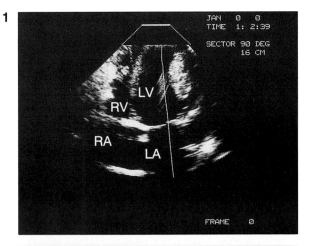

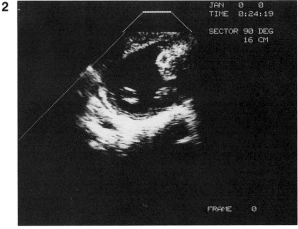

1 & 2 Echocardiographic appearance. LV, left ventricle; LA, left atrium; RV, right ventricle; RA, right atrium.

Answers

A (1) shows a 2-dimensional echocardiogram from the apical four-chamber view while (2) shows a similar image but from the parasternal short axis view. The left ventricular cavity is dilated and there is a large echogenic mass adherent to the left ventricular free wall. There are lucent areas visible within the echogenic mass (best seen in the parasternal short axis view). Furthermore, there is a smaller but similar mass visible in the right ventricular cavity and this appeared very mobile on real-time imaging. The echocardiographic appearance are is consistent with intracardiac (mural) thrombi in dilated left and right ventricles.

B While the shortness of breath could be due to left ventricular dysfunction the presence of mural thrombus raises a strong possibility of pulmonary embolism. Arterial blood gas analysis was performed and revealed arterial hypoxaemia and hypocapnia, and a ventilation/perfusion isotope lung scan was requested. This showed large segmental perfusion defects in the presence of a normal ventilation scan, making a pulmonary embolus very likely (3). The patient was, therefore, commenced on intravenous heparin with careful monitoring of the activated partial thromboplastin time (twice control value). Warfarin was later initiated and recommended as probable lifelong treatment. The patient was also commenced on the angiotensin-converting enzyme inhibitor, enalapril, as a prophylaxis against progressive left ventricular dilatation and dysfunction.

Reference

Hunter S, Hall R. Echocardiography. In: *Diseases of the Heart*. Julian DG, Camm AJ, Fox KM, Hall RJC, Poole-Wilson PA. London: Baillière Tindall, 1989.

3

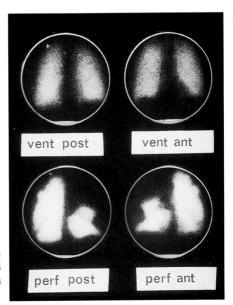

3 Ventilation (using $^{81}Kr^m$) and perfusion (using $^{99}Tc^M$) images. The perfusion (perf) scan reveals filling defects but the ventilation (vent) scan shows a normal distribution.

Index